Important Contact Information

MOM'S DOCTOR OR MIDWIFE: _____

_____

BIRTH DOULA: _____

_____

BABY'S DOCTOR: _____

_____

LACTATION CONSULTANT: _____

_____

LA LECHE LEADER: _____

_____

NEW MOTHERS' GROUP FACILITATOR: _____

_____

DAYCARE PROVIDER: _____

_____

POISON CONTROL CENTER: _____

_____

THE
EXPECTANT
PARENTS'
COMPANION

· ·

SIMPLIFYING WHAT TO DO,
BUY, OR BORROW FOR AN
EASY LIFE WITH BABY

Kathleen Huggins, R.N., M.S.

THE HARVARD COMMON PRESS · BOSTON, MASSACHUSETTS

The Harvard Common Press
535 Albany Street
Boston, Massachusetts 02118
www.harvardcommonpress.com

Printed in the United States of America
Printed on acid-free paper

Library of Congress Cataloging-in-Publication Data
Huggins, Kathleen.
  The expectant parents' companion : simplifying what to do, buy, or
borrow for an easy life with baby / Kathleen Huggins.
      p. cm.
  Includes index.
  ISBN 1-55832-333-3 (hardcover : alk. paper) — ISBN 1-55832-
334-1 (pbk. : alk. paper)
  1. Infants—Care. 2. Infants' supplies. 3. Pregnant women—Life
skills guide. 4. Pregnancy—Popular works. 5. Childbirth—Popular
works. I. Title.
  RJ61.H894 2006
  649'.122—dc22

                                                    2005031507

ISBN-13: 978-1-55832-333-9 (hardcover); 978-1-55832-334-6
(paperback)
ISBN-10: 1-55832-333-3 (hardcover); 1-55832-334-1 (paperback)

Special bulk-order discounts are available on this and other Harvard
Common Press books. Companies and organizations may purchase
books for premiums or resale, or may arrange a custom edition, by
contacting the Marketing Director at the address above.

Cover design by Night & Day Design
Interior design by Barbara Balch

10 9 8 7 6 5 4 3 2 1

To my husband, Brad

Contents

· ·

Introduction

. . . .

THE EXPECTANT PARENTS' COMPANION is a concise, straightforward guide to getting ready for life with your newborn. My aim is to provide all the essential information that new parents need—about childbirth classes, labor assistants, and baby doctors; about how to write and use a birth plan; about the best parenting books for the home library; about diapering, feeding the baby, selecting daycare, and baby-proofing the home. This book also tells what you need to know before buying baby gear.

"Baby gear?" my grandmother might have asked. She didn't own even a crib for my mother, who slept through her infancy in a dresser drawer. But the average low- to middle-income family with a baby born this year will spend $200,000 to $300,000 over the course of that child's first eighteen years, college costs excluded. Even before a baby is born, many parents spend thousands of dollars on baby-care equipment.

Today's parents have a dizzying array of gear from which to choose, much of it expensive. Over the past two decades there has been an explosion of new equipment for babies. Until you walk down the aisles of a baby "superstore," you can't imagine how many variations there can be on the same basic products. Car seats, cribs, strollers, and devices you never heard of are marketed with ever-newer "must-have" features. Promising safety, ease, style, and sometimes even a smarter baby, these products and their special features are sold as necessities.

Pressure to buy this stuff comes not only from retailers and parenting magazines but also from friends and family. Parents-to-be want to do things perfectly, and many assume this means having all of the best baby equipment. A pregnant belly seems to require a spending spree.

You might ask parents you know whether they bought any baby things that they ended up not using. You will hear about items that failed to work well, that the baby disliked, or that the family simply found few occasions to use. Because most new parents don't know better and are lured by marketers' hype, nearly all have bought unnecessary baby things.

Before you go shopping for baby gear, *The Expectant Parents' Companion* can help you sort out which items are truly helpful, which are useful for only a short time, and which may actually be dangerous. The book will help you figure out which products you really want to own, which you should borrow, and when you need to get them. By simplifying the choices for you, this book will help you resist pressure to spend a lot of money, fill your house with colored plastic stuff, and rely on various devices for holding and entertaining your baby.

This book may save you, for example, from spending as much as $100 on a swiveling "activity center" or "stationary entertainer" in which to stand the baby. Devised after baby walkers were pronounced dangerous, these bulky contraptions tend to bore babies and, if overused, may even delay a child's development, according to researchers.

Today there is a booming business, too, in safety gadgets—every imaginable sort for every potential danger. Naturally anxious and protective, new parents may be inclined to overspend on safety gear. Although every home should be checked for hazards, the best protection for a baby is careful supervision and common sense. If you feel the bath water before putting the baby into it, you can probably get along fine without a bathtub thermometer.

Throughout modern times, parenting philosophies have gone in and out of style. Now we're in a period of opposite extremes, from strict feeding and sleeping schedules to all-day baby "wearing" and all-night bed-sharing. What kind of baby gear you'll use—and how much of it—depends on how you want to raise your child. If you anticipate raising your baby very differently from the way you were raised, you may not totally trust the advice of family or friends. You may not even be sure which baby-rearing practices you favor. You may have strong opinions about pacifiers, disposable diapers, and cribs, or you may have no clue whether you will use these things.

Remember this: However much baby-care methods and equipment change, the basic needs of infants stay the same. Babies want loving attention, a mother's breast, and near constant contact. The best products on the market are those that help meet these needs. But many of the products available are just substitutes for the things that parents give. Swings and bouncers take the place of a parent's arms. Bottles take the place of the breast. Playpens take the place of a sharp eye, and strollers the place of a comfortable hip or a strong back. What this means is that to meet your baby's needs best you need purchase very little. If you nurse your baby instead of feeding formula, if you carry your baby until he is able to walk, and if you launder a couple of dozen cloth diapers instead of buying box after box of disposables, you can truly get by with very little, and you can be sure your baby will be content. Modern ideas and fancy equipment often just complicate and clutter families' lives.

With good, basic information and faith in your own intuition, you can raise your baby into a happy, healthy child while conserving resources—your own and the planet's—and staying happier yourself as well.

CHAPTER I

To Do and To Get

These checklists will help you start getting organized for your baby's arrival. The "To-do Checklist" is divided into four sections, for mid-pregnancy, the last trimester, late pregnancy, and after the birth. The "To-buy-or-borrow Checklist," also divided into time periods, shows you at a glance which baby items you really need, which ones are optional, and when the best time is to acquire various things. For more information about particular recommendations, consult the pages indicated.

TO-DO CHECKLIST

. . . .

MID-PREGNANCY

☐ Check your insurance plan for details on coverage of prenatal care, delivery, and hospitalization.

☐ Tour and choose a hospital where you plan to have the baby.

☐ Preregister at the hospital.

☐ Sign up for prenatal classes (see page 12).

☐ Read books about pregnancy and childbirth (see page 141).

☐ Begin writing your birth plan (see page 13).

☐ Interview doulas if you plan to hire one for labor or post-partum help (see page 19).

☐ Register at a store for preferred baby gifts.

☐ If you will be returning to work, start researching child-care options.

THIRD TRIMESTER

☐ Attend prenatal classes.

☐ Hire a labor assistant (doula), if you plan to use one.

☐ Complete your birth plan.

☐ Start planning the nursery, if you intend to have one.

☐ Purchase or borrow baby furniture, clothes, diapers, and other gear, including a car seat.

☐ Make sure your baby will be covered by medical insurance.

☐ Consider purchasing life insurance for yourself.

☐ Consider creating or updating your will or trust.

☐ Interview and choose a baby doctor (see page 20).

☐ Decide whether or not you'll breastfeed.

☐ Decide whether you'll have your son circumcised.

☐ Buy bottle-feeding supplies, if you plan on formula feeding.

☐ If you'll use a diaper service, sign up.

☐ Discuss your parental-leave plan with your employer.

☐ Choose birth announcements and thank-you notes.

☐ Post an emergency-contact list near the phone.

☐ Start baby-proofing your home.

☐ Identify breastfeeding support, including a lactation consultant and a source for renting an electric pump.

☐ Consider baby names.

LATE PREGNANCY

☐ If you've had a baby shower, write thank-you notes.

☐ If you will need child-care help, interview providers (see page 131).

☐ Pack a suitcase for the hospital stay or assemble home-birth supplies.

☐ Practice breathing and other relaxation techniques with your partner.

☐ Review your birthing plan with your doctor or midwife.

☐ Buy nursing bras, if needed, and other breastfeeding supplies such as nursing pads and lanolin (see page 30).

☐ Install the car seat and have an expert check the installation (see page 90).

☐ Wash all of the baby clothes and bedding.

☐ Arrange for helpers for the first week or two after delivery (see page 24).

☐ Get the names of postpartum support groups (see page 25).

☐ Prepare and freeze several meals for the first couple of weeks at home.

☐ Read about breastfeeding and baby care.

☐ Consider a small gift for the hospital staff.

☐ Get a haircut.

AFTER DELIVERY

- ☐ Rest when the baby sleeps.

- ☐ Notify your insurance company about your baby's birth.

- ☐ Apply for and get a copy of your baby's birth certificate.

- ☐ Apply for a Social Security number for the baby.

- ☐ Buy or rent a breast pump if you will need one (see page 32).

- ☐ Borrow or buy other baby gear as you think you need it.

- ☐ Send birth announcements.

- ☐ Schedule a first doctor's visit for your baby and a postpartum checkup for Mom.

- ☐ Continue baby-proofing your home (see page 121).

TO-BUY-OR-BORROW CHECKLIST

. . . .

EARLY TO MID-PREGNANCY

☐ Books about pregnancy, childbirth, and baby care
(see The Parenting Bookshelf, page 141)

☐ Maternity clothes

MID-PREGNANCY THROUGH THE EIGHTH MONTH

☐ Car seat (see page 90)

☐ Dresser (see page 65)

☐ Baby bed (cradle, bassinet, bedside sleeper, or crib;
see page 57)

☐ Layette items (see page 68)

☐ Diapers (cloth or disposable; see page 72)

☐ Baby-care supplies (see page 78)

☐ Bottle-feeding supplies, if you plan to use them
(see page 47)

☐ Initial baby-proofing supplies (see page 121)

☐ Diaper bag (see page 107)

☐ Soft cloth carrier (see page 95)

Optional Items (in addition to those already listed)

☐ *Bassinet (see page 58)*

☐ *Cradle (see page 57)*

☐ *Play yard with or without bassinet (see page 59)*

☐ *Bedside sleeper (see page 58)*

☐ *Changing table (see page 64)*

☐ *Rocking chair or glider (see page 65)*

☐ *Electronic baby monitor (see page 66)*

☐ *Stroller (see page 100)*

EARLY IN THE NINTH MONTH

☐ Nursing bras and other breastfeeding supplies, if needed (see page 30)

☐ Waterproof mattress cover (see page 25)

☐ Postpartum supplies (see page 23)

☐ Birth supplies for a hospital delivery (see page 22)

FIRST TWO MONTHS AFTER THE BIRTH

☐ Breast pump, if needed (see page 32)

Optional Items (in addition to those already listed)

☐ *Bouncer seat (see page 84)*

☐ *Baby swing (see page 85)*

FOUR TO SIX MONTHS AFTER THE BIRTH

☐ High chair and feeding supplies (see page 111)

☐ Baby-proofing supplies (see page 121)

Optional Items (in addition to those already listed)

☐ *Crib (see page 59)*

☐ *Frame backpack (see page 98)*

☐ *Stationary entertainer (see page 86)*

CHAPTER 2

Preparing for Your Baby's Birth

One of the keys to getting off to a good start caring for your baby is to have an uncomplicated birth. Although medically managed birth is now the norm in the United States, parents—and society—may pay a higher price for it than most people know.

PLAN FOR AN UNCOMPLICATED BIRTH

. . . .

Most new mothers today opt for epidural anesthesia. They make this choice mainly out of fear—the fear of pain in childbirth. But ignorance is a factor, too. No one may tell a woman that having an epidural means being confined to bed, with an intravenous drip, a catheter to the bladder, and straps across the belly to monitor the baby's heart rate continuously. No one may tell her that epidurals often slow labor, in which case a woman is given synthetic oxytocin (Pitocin) to speed contractions, or that the intense contractions brought on by Pitocin can cause a drop in blood pressure, which can in turn deprive the baby of oxygen. Nobody may say that epidural anesthesia sometimes causes, in both mother and baby, a fever that must be treated with antibiotics, or that after epidural anesthesia a woman may itch all over. No one may say that an epidural reduces a woman's ability to push, so that the doctor may have to pull the baby out with forceps or a vacuum extractor. And no one may tell a woman that if she accepts epidural anesthesia for her first labor she increases by two to three times her risk of ending up with a cesarean.

Besides the temptation of anesthesia, another hazard for women approaching labor is the seduction of induction. When a woman nears or passes her due date and grows tired of being pregnant, her doctor may suggest inducing labor, usually by breaking the bag of waters, at a time convenient for both doctor and client. Hurrying the onset of labor this way often results in a very long labor, the use of Pitocin to speed contractions, and, finally, birth by cesarean.

When the baby arrives, a woman who has had a complicated, anesthetized, or cesarean birth is likely to experience more troubles. She may be separated from the baby. She may have difficulty starting to breastfeed. Her milk may take longer to come in. Her recovery may take longer, and she may have a hard time caring for the baby for several weeks after birth.

Sometimes problems arising naturally in labor make medical intervention necessary. But a woman who chooses medication or induction is inviting a cascade of interventions that may have been entirely unnecessary. She loses control of what happens to her and her newborn, and she ends up unhappy. So if you want a satisfying birth experience and a peaceful postpartum period, start by choosing natural birth.

VISIT THE HOSPITAL OR BIRTH CENTER

You have probably already selected a doctor or midwife, but you may have other choices yet to make about the birth, including, perhaps, the place. Your doctor or midwife may have privileges at more than one facility and may even attend home births. Your insurance plan may also give you options. To compare facilities, or to make the best of whatever is available to you, you will want to educate yourself a bit more about birthing practices; see the list of "Best Books about Birth" on the next page. Then, if you plan to deliver at a hospital or birth center, take a tour. On your tour, ask some of these questions:

THE BASICS:
- How many laboring women is each nurse assigned to?
- Are birth plans welcomed (see page 13)?
- How many family members or other people are allowed in the birth room?
- Are professional labor assistants welcome (see page 19)?
- Are photographs permitted?

IF YOU WOULD PREFER A NATURAL BIRTH:
- How are contractions and fetal heart tones monitored in labor? (With a Doppler ultrasound stethoscope or with an

electronic fetal monitor? If the latter, is the monitoring intermittent, continuous, or by telemetry (wireless monitoring? External or internal?)

◆ Are women free to move about in labor?

◆ Is the use of a shower, bathtub, or birthing pool permitted?

◆ What comfort devices are available, such as a birthing ball or birthing chair?

◆ Are eating and drinking allowed during labor?
   (Some hospitals allow women only to suck on ice chips.)

IF YOU'RE CONSIDERING A MEDICATED BIRTH:

◆ What choices other than epidural anesthesia are available for pain management?

◆ Is it possible to have an epidural that is light enough to allow moving in bed?

IF YOU ARE PLANNING A CESAREAN BIRTH:

◆ Are support persons welcome in the room during the delivery?

INFANT CARE AFTER A VAGINAL BIRTH:

◆ Can the mother hold the baby against her skin during the initial evaluation?

◆ Can weighing, bathing, and routine medications be delayed for the first hour or two?

◆ Is early breastfeeding encouraged?

◆ Can the mother's partner bathe the baby?

INFANT CARE AFTER A CESAREAN BIRTH:

◆ How much contact can the mother have with the baby immediately after the birth?

◆ Can the partner accompany the baby to the nursery?

◆ Can the baby be returned to the mother in the recovery room?

◆ Is early breastfeeding encouraged?

BEST BOOKS ABOUT BIRTH

For more information about these books, see The Parenting Bookshelf, page 141.

Pregnancy, Childbirth, and the Newborn: The Complete Guide, rev. ed., by Penny Simkin, Janet Whalley, and Ann Keppler

The Birth Partner: Everything You Need to Know to Help a Woman Through Childbirth, 2nd ed., by Penny Simkin

Active Birth: The New Approach to Giving Birth Naturally, rev. ed., by Janet Balaskas

The Official Lamaze Guide: Giving Birth with Confidence, by Judith Lothian and Charlotte DeVries

POSTPARTUM CARE:

◆ What is a typical hospital stay following a vaginal or cesarean birth? Is it possible to leave the hospital early?

◆ Are mothers allowed to keep their babies with them around the clock?

◆ If a baby is in the nursery, is he brought to the mother whenever he seems hungry? Are newborns routinely offered water or formula after nursings or while in the nursery?

◆ Is a lactation consultant on staff for breastfeeding assistance?

◆ Has the hospital received or applied for certification as a UNICEF Baby-Friendly Hospital? (This would signify that the hospital's policies promote breastfeeding.)

If you'd like to give birth at home, you'll need a practitioner—probably a midwife—who attends home births, and your pregnancy will have to be "low-risk" and healthy. You'll want to ask the midwife these questions:

◆ Does she have hospital admitting privileges and a backup physician, in case of emergency?

◆ Will she provide labor support if you are admitted to the hospital?

◆ Does she have a backup midwife in case she is unavailable when you go into labor?

◆ What resuscitative equipment does she bring to the home?

TAKE A CLASS OR TWO

If you haven't had a baby before, you will definitely benefit from a prepared-childbirth class. In it you'll learn how labor and delivery happen, how to develop a birth plan, how to work as a team in labor, and how to relax when labor begins. If you are still in the first or second trimester, you might also sign up for an early-pregnancy class. For later in the pregnancy, you might check whether your hospital or another local organization offers classes in cesarean preparation, breastfeeding, baby care, or CPR.

Early-Pregnancy Classes

These classes are often taught by obstetrical nurses. Topics include the physical and emotional changes of early pregnancy, coping with symptoms of pregnancy, fetal growth and development, and maternal nutrition and exercise.

Prepared-Childbirth Classes

These classes are typically intended for the last trimester, but you may need to sign up earlier to get a place. Classes offered by hospitals and birth centers are usually free to prospective clients. Private classes taught by certified instructors are generally smaller and well worth their cost. Before you sign up for a class, ask what it covers, and ask about the instructor's credentials. You might even ask her for a reference or two.

Most prepared-childbirth teachers follow one of three systems of instruction:

LAMAZE. The most popular prepared-childbirth method in the United States, Lamaze teaches relaxation, breathing, and focusing techniques to help women manage the discomforts of labor. Lamaze classes are geared toward promoting, protecting, and supporting normal birth. A typical course has six sessions. To find a certified Lamaze instructor in your area, call 800-368-4404.

BRADLEY. The originator of the idea of husbands as childbirth "coaches," the Bradley method also teaches about nutrition in pregnancy and breathing and relaxation in labor. Bradley classes are geared toward unmedicated birth. A course usually includes twelve sessions. To find a Bradley instructor in your area, call 800-4-A-BIRTH.

INTERNATIONAL CHILDBIRTH EDUCATION ASSOCIATION (ICEA). Since this organization doesn't promote any particular childbirth method, courses taught by ICEA-certified teachers vary greatly in structure and content. But all ICEA teachers believe that maternity care should be centered around families' needs and desires rather than the routines of hospital staff. To find an ICEA-certified instructor in your area, call 952-854-8660.

MAKE A BIRTH PLAN

After you have learned about the policies and typical procedures at the hospital or birth center you've chosen, and after you have completed most or all of your childbirth classes, you will be ready to write up your preferences in a birth plan. Your birth plan tells the nursing staff and your primary caregiver what you would like for your labor, delivery, and postpartum care.

Your plan doesn't have to be comprehensive. For example, unless enemas and shaving of pubic hair are routine at the hospital, you don't need to request an exemption from these procedures. (Of course, if you do need an exemption from such routines—and, especially, from rules requiring confinement to bed and an IV— you may want to consider giving birth somewhere else.) Keep your plan simple and clear. Page after page of requests will probably go unread. Focus on what you really care about.

Don't let your plan sound like a list of demands. Instead of "I do not want an episiotomy" (a cut through the perineum), say, "I hope to avoid an episiotomy." Be positive. Issues you may want to consider include:

◆ Support persons

◆ Movements or positions you may use

◆ Interventions, such as fetal monitoring, artificial rupture of the membranes, and episiotomy

◆ Keeping hydrated (by sipping drinks, sucking ice chips, or having an IV)

◆ Pain relief (massage, hot and cold packs, relaxation and breathing exercises, use of a tub or shower, medication)

◆ Baby care, including feeding and keeping the baby in your room

Examples of specific requests are listed in the following pages, Guidelines for Your Birth Plan.

Once you have written your birth plan, schedule time to review it with both your doctor or midwife and the baby's doctor so that you can make sure the plan is realistic and will be respected. Afterward, make copies of the plan for your caregiver, for the hospital staff, for the baby's doctor, and for your partner or professional labor assistant.

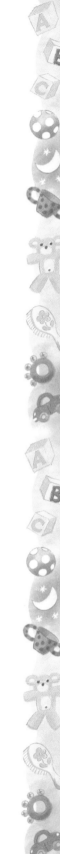

GUIDELINES FOR

Your Birth Plan

LABOR SUPPORT

☐ A doula as well as my partner will be present during the labor and birth.

LABOR PREFERENCES

☐ I wish to be able to move around and change positions throughout labor.

☐ I would like to be able to drink throughout the first stage of labor.

☐ I would like to use a birthing chair/birthing ball/birthing pool/bathtub/shower during labor.

☐ We will bring a birthing chair/birthing ball/birthing pool.

☐ We will bring recorded music and a CD/tape player.

☐ We would like the room kept as quiet as possible.

☐ We would like the lights kept low.

☐ I would prefer to keep the number of vaginal exams to a minimum.

☐ Unless I become dehydrated, I wish to avoid an IV.

☐ I would like to wear my contact lenses/glasses at all times.

FETAL MONITORING

☐ I would prefer intermittent wireless rather than continuous fetal monitoring.

☐ I would prefer external to internal monitoring unless the baby shows signs of distress.

YOUR BIRTH PLAN, continued

INDUCTION AND AUGMENTATION OF LABOR

☐ I wish to have the membranes left intact until they break naturally, unless signs of fetal distress require internal monitoring.

☐ If labor is not progressing, I would prefer to try natural methods of speeding labor (position changes, walking, nipple stimulation) before the amniotic membrane is broken or Pitocin is administered.

☐ If labor is not progressing, I would like to try having the amniotic membrane broken before Pitocin is used.

PAIN MEDICATIONS

☐ I will request pain medication if I need it.

☐ Before considering an epidural, I would like to try narcotic pain relief.

☐ I would like to have a standard epidural.

☐ I would like to have a light epidural, so that I can move in bed.

CESAREAN BIRTH

☐ I would like to avoid a cesarean if at all possible.

☐ I would like to participate in decisions regarding a cesarean.

☐ If I have a cesarean, I would like my partner to be present.

☐ I would like my doula to be present.

☐ I would like the screen lowered just before the delivery so I can watch my baby's birth.

☐ Unless my baby needs urgent care, I would like to see him right after birth.

☐ Unless the baby needs urgent care, I would like my partner to hold him right after birth and to take him to the nursery.

☐ I would like the baby brought to the recovery room so I can hold him against my skin and start breastfeeding him.

EPISIOTOMY

☐ I hope to avoid an episiotomy unless it is needed for the baby's safety.

☐ I would prefer a small tear over an episiotomy.

DELIVERY

☐ I would like to choose the position (such as squatting or on hands and knees) in which I give birth.

☐ I would like a mirror available so I can see the baby's birth.

☐ I would like the chance to touch the baby's head when it crowns.

☐ Assuming the baby is not in distress, I would like to wait until I feel the urge to push.

☐ We would like to have the room as quiet as possible and the lights turned low for the actual delivery.

☐ I would like to hold the baby against my chest, skin to skin, as soon as he is born.

☐ We would like to photograph/videotape the birth.

YOUR BIRTH PLAN, continued

IMMEDIATELY AFTER DELIVERY

☐ I would prefer that the umbilical cord stop pulsating before it is cut.

☐ I would like to have my partner cut the cord.

☐ We would like to hold the baby for at least an hour before he is weighed, bathed, or examined.

☐ I would like to hold the baby while he is examined.

☐ I would like the baby to be examined and bathed in my room.

☐ I would like assistance as needed in putting the baby to breast in the first hour after delivery.

☐ If the baby seems chilled, I would like to warm him against my skin instead of having him wrapped and placed under heat lamps.

☐ I would like to delay eye medication for two hours following the birth.

☐ If the baby must be taken from me for medical treatment, I would like my partner to stay with the baby.

POSTPARTUM CARE

☐ I would prefer a private room.

☐ I would like to keep my baby with me 24 hours a day unless he must be observed in the nursery for medical reasons.

☐ I would like the baby with me during the day and evening but in the nursery at night.

☐ I would prefer the baby be kept in the nursery except when I ask for him or when he is hungry.

☐ I would like to breastfeed day and night, whenever the baby seems hungry.

☐ I wish the baby to receive a bottle only if medically necessary.

☐ I prefer that the baby not be given a pacifier.

☐ I would like to meet with a lactation consultant before discharge.

CONSIDER A PROFESSIONAL LABOR ASSISTANT

Many expectant parents now seek out the services of a professional labor assistant. Such a person may call herself a doula (from the Greek, "one who ministers") or a labor coach. She doesn't take over the partner's role of helping the mother; instead, the doula uses her extensive experience with labor to advise and assist both the mother and her partner, and she facilitates communication with the medical staff.

If you'd like to hire a labor assistant, you can ask your doctor, midwife, or childbirth educator for a referral (your childbirth educator may even work as a doula herself). Or you can call either of three organizations that provide training and certification for doulas: Childbirth and Postpartum Professional Association, 888-MY-CAPPA, Doulas of North America, 888-788-DONA, and the International Childbirth Education Association, 952-854-8660.

When you interview a labor assistant, ask about:

◆ Her training and certification

◆ Her references (names and phone numbers of other new parents she has helped)

◆ Her fee

◆ Her substitute in case she is unavailable

◆ A prenatal meeting to discuss your birth plan and her philosophy about childbirth

◆ Where and when she'll meet you during labor

FIND A BABY DOCTOR

Choosing a doctor you trust for your baby is one of your most important tasks during pregnancy.

Your baby's doctor will probably examine the baby in the hospital, will give him regular checkups and immunizations throughout infancy and beyond, and will serve as your adviser on your baby's health and development.

The doctor may be a pediatrician or a family physician. Also known as general practitioners, family physicians can serve the whole family, referring to specialists when necessary.

You can get the names of baby doctors from friends, from the hospital, or from your doctor or midwife. Since many doctors offer free get-acquainted visits, you may want to visit more than one. You will need to make sure that the doctor you choose is covered by your insurance plan and has privileges at the hospital where you plan to give birth. You may want to limit your choice of doctors to those with offices close to your home.

When you visit the doctor's office, pay attention to the nurse. This is generally the person who returns phone calls and responds to new parents' ordinary concerns. Is the nurse friendly and receptive to your questions?

A TYPICAL SCHEDULE FOR

Well-baby Exams

2 to 4 days	4 months*	15 months*
1 month	6 months*	18 months*
2 months*	12 months*	2 years*

Includes vaccinations

It may be a bonus if the physician employs a pediatric nurse practitioner. These nurses have special training in well-baby care. They may do checkups just as a physician does, but they usually spend more time talking with new parents.

Discuss with the doctor matters that are important to you, such as circumcision, sleep schedules, breastfeeding, and immunizations. A question like "What is your approach to breastfeeding problems?" will elicit more helpful information than "How do you feel about breastfeeding?"

Some practices employ their own lactation consultants. At a minimum, the doctor should be prepared to refer you to a local lactation consultant rather than recommending formula. Review with the doctor any elements of your birth plan that may require the doctor's special orders. You may need the doctor's approval to delay the baby's exam and bath until after the first nursing, to avoid routine supplemental bottles or a pacifier, or even to keep your baby in your hospital room around the clock.

If you are planning a home birth, find out whether the doctor will come to your home or, if not, when you should bring the baby in to the doctor's office.

Well-baby checkups are most frequent in infancy, when a baby develops very rapidly. The first is usually when the baby is two to four days old. Plan on about seven well-baby visits in the first year and three in the second. Each visit includes a physical examination and comparison with normal developmental milestones. Some visits may include hearing, vision, and other tests.

Most well-baby visits will include immunizations. These are controversial. You may want to read *The Immunization Resource Guide: Where to Find Answers to All Your Questions about Childhood Immunizations*, by Diane Rozario (see The Parenting Bookshelf, page 143).

ASSEMBLE SUPPLIES FOR THE BIRTH

For a hospital birth, you'll want to pack many of the following items.

FOR LABOR

- Insurance information and preregistration forms
- Your birth plan
- Eyeglasses or contact lenses
- A still or video camera and, if needed, film
- Massage lotion or oil
- Massager (could be a tennis ball, rolling pin, or full can of soda)
- Portable CD or tape player, and relaxing recordings
- Special picture
- Lip balm
- Suckers or other hard candy, in case your mouth gets dry
- Birthing ball
- Birthing pool, if you want to labor in water and the hospital permits it

- Important phone numbers, and phone card or plenty of change (some hospitals forbid the use of cell phones)
- Comfortable pillow
- Socks
- Champagne or sparkling cider (if the hospital doesn't provide it) to celebrate the birth

FOR THE PARTNER

- Underwear and shirt
- Bathing suit, for joining Mom in the birthing pool or shower
- Toothbrush
- Snacks
- Book, magazine, cards, games

FOR AFTER THE BIRTH

- Two or three nightgowns, with front access for nursing, or pairs of pajamas
- Robe and slippers
- Two or three nursing bras and sets of nursing pads
- 3 to 5 pairs underpants
- Toiletries: toothbrush, toothpaste, shampoo, hairbrush, etc. (most hospitals have blow dryers)
- Nursing pillow
- Small tube of lanolin, for tender nipples

FOR GOING HOME

- An outfit for yourself (something that fit you when you were five or six months pregnant)
- Extra-absorbent sanitary pads with wings
- An outfit for the baby, including an undershirt, a receiving blanket, and a hat
- An empty bag, for hospital giveaways
- A car seat, installed in the car

ARRANGE FOR HELP FOR AFTER THE BIRTH

The period of several weeks after birth is a time for rest, recovery, and learning how to feed and comfort your newborn. To avoid physical and mental exhaustion, you'll want to set very minimal goals for yourself each day and to nap or rest whenever the baby sleeps. You'll need plenty of help to manage this. Welcome assistance from other people with household chores and meals. Invite friends and family members to do laundry, care for the lawn or garden, watch the baby while you nap, or bring over a hot dish.

Sometimes you may find yourself just needing someone to talk to. Again, reach out to friends and family. Your doctor or midwife, your baby's doctor, and a lactation consultant or volunteer breastfeeding counselor may also be helpful when you need advice and reassurance.

If friends and family are less available than you need, consider hiring a postpartum doula. She can help with breastfeeding and baby care, do light housekeeping, run errands, and prepare meals. Ask your doctor, midwife, or childbirth educator for a referral, call one of three national doula organizations, or visit their Web sites:

Childbirth and Postpartum Professional Association, 888-MY-CAPPA, www.cappa.net

Doulas of North America, 888-788-DONA, www.dona.org

National Association of Postpartum Care Services, 800-453-6852, www.napcs.org

More expensive than a doula is a baby nurse. This is not a medical nurse but someone who has made a career out of caring for newborns. Baby nurses come into the home to care for a baby from 6 to 24 hours per day. They do not assist with any other duties in the home. More practical than hiring a baby nurse may be arranging for a cleaning service, to keep the house tidy while you care for the baby.

PREPARATIONS FOR

The First Weeks After Birth

◆ Arrange for help from friends, family, a doula, or a housekeeper.

◆ Plan to nap when the baby does.

◆ Get a waterproof pad to protect your mattress from postpartum bleeding and sweating and from leaking milk.

◆ Prepare soups, stews, and casseroles for the freezer.

◆ Stock up on high-energy foods that won't spoil quickly, such as eggs, peanut butter, cereal, juice, nuts, and dried fruits.

◆ Get the name and phone number of a local lactation consultant.

◆ Get the names and phone numbers of new-mothers' support groups.

When you feel ready to go out, you may want to attend a meeting of a new-mothers' support group such as those offered by La Leche League. You can learn about local groups from your doctor or midwife, your baby's doctor, your childbirth educator, your lactation consultant, or even your phone book. If your family income is low, you might investigate whether you qualify for the WIC (Women, Infants, and Children) Supplemental Food Program, which is available in every state. WIC provides food for breastfeeding women, formula coupons for babies who are bottle-fed, and nutritional counseling for breastfeeding and infancy. You can find a phone number for WIC in the governmental pages of your local phone directory or get it from your county health department.

CHAPTER 3

Getting Ready for Breastfeeding

Breastfeeding is best for all babies' health and development. Mother's milk is uniquely designed to meet the complete nutritional needs of growing babies and to protect them against illness throughout the nursing period and beyond.

Breastfeeding is economical, too. Nursing a baby through her first year saves $1,200 to $4,000 in formula costs, and perhaps much more in medical care and lost work time, because breastfed babies get sick less often than formula-fed babies.

LEARN ABOUT BREASTFEEDING

. . . .

Nursing is a skill that a mother and her baby must learn together in the first weeks after birth. Often this isn't easy. It helps to study ahead by taking a breastfeeding class (see page 12), reading about breastfeeding, and attending a La Leche League meeting or two to get a close-up view of early nursing (see page 146). Having the name and number of a local lactation consultant is important, too, in case you need hands-on help when nursing begins.

A FEW REASONS

Breastfeeding Is Better

Compared with formula-fed babies:

♦ Breastfed babies experience less sickness and hospitalization from diarrhea, respiratory infections, and ear infections.

♦ Breastfed babies experience fewer urinary-tract infections and fewer cases of bacterial meningitis.

♦ Breastfed babies are less likely to succumb to Sudden Infant Death Syndrome.

♦ Breastfed babies are less likely to suffer tooth decay in early childhood.

♦ Breastfed babies are less likely to experience learning disorders and intellectual impairment as they grow up.

♦ Breastfed babies are less likely to become obese in adulthood.

The most important skill to master is getting the baby latched on to the breast, so that she drains it effectively and does not injure the nipple. Women don't know instinctively how to do this. You can learn techniques for correct positioning from a breastfeeding class or from *The Nursing Mother's Companion* (see The Parenting Bookshelf, page 141).

BEST BOOK ABOUT BREASTFEEDING

The Nursing Mother's Companion, 5th ed., by Kathleen Huggins

PURCHASES
TO CONSIDER

. . . .

Breastfeeding requires no equipment besides what nature provides. Still, there are a few things you might want to buy to make nursing your baby easier.

In the early weeks, breastfeeding is usually most comfortable in an armchair. Sitting up straight can be difficult on a couch or bed, and it's important to sit up straight while learning to position the baby correctly. You may already have a chair in your home that will be perfect; if not, you might be able to borrow a chair or buy one used. If your home has two levels, you'll want to have two comfortable armchairs.

You don't need an ottoman to go with your chair. An inexpensive, wooden nursing footstool works much better (see Other Resources for New Parents, page 146).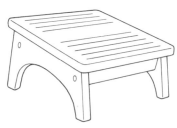

Nursing bras aren't an absolute necessity, but they provide good support and, usually through cups that unhook at the top, easy access to the breasts. The best time to buy nursing bras is during the last two to three weeks of pregnancy, when the breasts are closest to their maximum size. At this time the cups should fit a little loosely, since the breasts will get fuller when the milk comes in, about three days after the birth. The band should fit when attached on the outer row of hooks, because the rib cage will shrink somewhat after the birth. You may want to buy just two or three bras before the birth, so you can see which style works best before buying more. Whether or not the bras you buy are designed for nursing, they will be most comfortable if they have no underwires (which can cause plugged milk ducts and breast infections) and if they are made of cotton or microfiber, the most breathable fabrics.

You don't really need other special clothes for nursing, since any top that you can pull up from the bottom will work well. In the early weeks, though, the typical mom spends a great deal of time getting her baby latched on correctly, and she may feel quite exposed if she must do this with her shirt tucked under her chin. Special nursing clothes with slits in front help a new mom nurse more discreetly. Since many new mothers spend a lot of time in their nightwear in the early weeks, you might consider buying a nursing nightgown or pajama set. For going out, you may want a nursing top or two. Nursing clothes are sold at most maternity shops.

For women who leak milk, as most do in the early weeks, nursing pads keep the bra and shirt dry so they don't need washing as often. There are two basic kinds of nursing pads, washable and disposable. Washable pads, made of cloth, are more economical for women who leak

A nursing top

for several weeks or longer. Leaking colostrum in pregnancy is a sure sign that a woman will leak milk later. In this case, I recommend buying at least eight pairs of cloth pads before the birth. For women who don't leak in pregnancy, I recommend getting just one box of disposable pads in advance. Some women end up never using a pad, but being prepared may save an inconvenient run to the drugstore.

Lansinoh disposable pads are a favorite with nursing mothers. These pads are very thin and absorbent, with a wicking lining that keeps both the nipples and the bra dry. The pads are contoured to fit the breasts without puckers, and they come with adhesive tape to keep the pads in place. Lansinoh pads are available in drugstores (see Other Resources for New Parents, page 146). To save money, you can make your own nursing pads, cut out of diapers or toweling and stitched around the edge.

Since a new baby is too small to support on the mother's lap for nursing, a mom may find it helpful to place a pillow on her lap before positioning the baby. An ordinary bed pillow works well for this purpose, but today a variety of pillows are being marketed especially for nursing. Some of these, crescent-shaped to wrap around the body, were originally designed for training older babies to sit. These tend to create a gap between the pillow and the mother's body, and the baby tends to sink into the gap. Much better is a firm pillow with a flat surface to support the baby. By far the best of the commercial nursing pillows is My Brest Friend (see Other Resources for New Parents, page 146).

Another thing to have on hand before the birth is a small tube of medical-grade lanolin, which is available in many drugstores. Lanolin can't prevent sore nipples, but it can soothe them and promote their healing. Although some hospitals hand out lanolin to new mothers, others don't, so be sure to pack some in your hospital bag.

You don't need to buy or rent a breast pump before the birth, but if you haven't found a lactation consultant you might check into where you can rent a hospital-grade, fully automatic pump in case you have problems establishing breastfeeding. To locate a rental station near you, call either of the two manufacturers of these pumps, Medela (800-435-8316) or Hollister (800-323-4060). Once breastfeeding is established, you will want to pick a pump based on your needs. For a mother not planning to work away from home, a small pump may be adequate. Good models are made by Medela and Avent; most others are a waste of money. For a woman returning to full- or part-time work, buying a small, ineffective pump is a false economy; a high-end pump is needed for emptying the breast completely and thus maintaining high milk production. For descriptions of pump models available, consult *The Nursing Mother's Companion* (see The Parenting Bookshelf, page 141). Once you know which model you'd like to buy, shop around for the best price. High-end pumps are available for sale at some maternity and baby stores and from some lactation consultants.

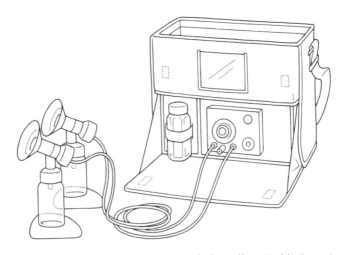

The best-selling Medela Pump-in-Style

Don't try to save money by borrowing another woman's pump. An unsterilized pump can transmit bacteria and viruses, and some pumps are difficult to sterilize.

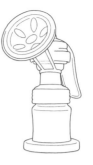

When you buy your pump, you may also want to buy a few bottles and nipples for feeding your baby your breast milk. For tips on buying bottles and nipples, see page 47. Avent bottles and nipples, available in drugstores and supermarkets, are favorites among

The hand-operated Avent Isis

nursing mothers. These nipples have various flow speeds, which are identified according to a baby's age.

You'll need plenty of bottles if you'll be pumping often and freezing the milk in the feeding bottles. Mother's Milk Mate is a

---

THINGS TO GET

For Breastfeeding

- ◆ Armchair (if you don't already have one)
- ◆ Nursing footstool (optional)
- ◆ Nursing bras (or other supportive bras without underwire)
- ◆ Nursing outerwear (optional)
- ◆ Nursing pads (cloth or disposable)
- ◆ Nursing pillow (optional)
- ◆ Tube of medical-grade lanolin
- ◆ Breast pump (wait until after the birth)
- ◆ Bottles, nipples, and storage bags (wait until after the birth)

BREASTFEEDING HELP

If your doctor or midwife, the baby's doctor, or your child-birth educator hasn't been able to identify a local lactation consultant for you, call Medela (800-435-8316) or Hollister (800-323-4060) for a referral. Or see the Web site for the International Lactation Consultant Association (www.ilca.org), which lists practicing lactation consultants by Zip Code.

---

nice freezer rack that comes with 10 bottles (see Other Resources for New Parents, page 146). Many women prefer to freeze their milk in special milk-storage bags into which many pumps allow direct pumping (see Other Resources for New Parents, page 146). These bags are available from lactation consultants and from some maternity and baby stores.

CHAPTER 4

Getting Ready for Formula Feeding

If you know that you or your partner won't be
able to breastfeed your baby and so must use formula instead, you have a lot to learn ahead of time.

First, you can't feed a baby on regular cow's
milk, goat's milk, soymilk, or rice milk—straight,
diluted, or mixed with other foods. No homemade
formula contains all of the nutrients a baby needs
to grow and stay healthy. If your baby isn't breastfed, he must have commercial formula throughout
his first year.

TYPES OF FORMULA

. . . .

Commercial formula comes in three forms: ready-to-feed, concentrate, and powdered. Both concentrated and powdered formula must be mixed with water. Ready-to-feed formula is most expensive; if you use it for a year, you'll spend at least $1,700. That's if you buy 32-ounce cans; if you buy it in 8-ounce cans, you'll spend as much as $4,000 for the year. Concentrate costs about $1,500 per year, powdered about $1,200 per year. Although powdered is cheapest, you shouldn't use it in your baby's first month; studies have found that over half of all cans of this formula are contaminated with salmonella or another member of its family (such as *Enterobacter sakazakii,* which can cause various deadly infections), and babies with very immature immune systems may be overcome by these microbes.

The most common formulas are made of cow's milk. Soy and "predigested" formulas are used for infants who can't tolerate cow's milk, although there are concerns about the high levels of aluminum in these formulas. Soy formula costs $1,300 to $2,000 for a baby's first year. "Predigested" formula, which is fed to babies who can't tolerate either cow's milk or soy, costs as much as $2,400 per year.

The American Academy of Pediatrics recommends that all formula fed to babies be fortified with iron. Although most formulas are, some cow's-milk formulas aren't. Iron-fortified formula helps prevent iron deficiency, the most common cause of anemia in children. Some physicians and parents, however, believe that iron-fortified formula causes colic symptoms, including constipation, diarrhea, spitting up, and vomiting. Numerous studies contradict this belief.

Only a few companies manufacture baby formula. Regardless of what your baby's doctor may tell you, there is little difference between brands. Generic formulas are fine, too.

EXPECT DISCOMFORT IN DRYING UP

After a woman gives birth, the loss of the placenta signals her body to begin making milk. Around the third day after birth, her breasts usually become swollen and tender as they fill with milk. This engorgement goes away by itself in a week or two if the mother doesn't breastfeed or pump her milk. In the meantime, a supportive bra, a mild pain reliever, and ice packs can help relieve the discomfort. Some lactation professionals also recommend the old remedy of chilled cabbage leaves worn inside the bra. It helps to express a little milk, but only a little, unless you want to prolong milk production.

Few doctors today prescribe "dry-up" medication, because these drugs can have serious side effects. They also take several days to work, and after a 10-day course of medication the breasts sometimes resume producing milk.

LEARN TO PREPARE FORMULA SAFELY

Unlike breast milk, formula contains no antibodies or other constituents that protect babies from disease. Because of this, and because a newborn's own immune system has little ability to fight infection, you'll want to be very careful to avoid introducing germs when you prepare formula and feed it to your baby. Sterilizing bottles, nipples, and formula for your baby's first four months will help keep him safe from gastrointestinal illness.

Just as important as using sterile technique is careful attention to directions. These vary from brand to brand and may change occasionally for any particular brand, so read the directions that come with each container of formula that you buy. Overdiluting formula can stunt a baby's growth; underdiluting formula can burden his kidneys and digestive system and lead to dehydration. Here are some general rules to ensure accurate measurement:

◆ When using powdered formula, use the measuring scoop that comes with the formula.

◆ Don't shake or tap the scoop; level the powder with the flat edge of a knife.

◆ When measuring water or liquid concentrate, use a clear glass measuring cup. Your eyes should be level with the top of the liquid as you check the measurement.

There are four methods for sterilizing formula and feeding equipment: the aseptic method, the terminal sterilization method, and two single-bottle methods. These are described on pages 39 to 42. Any of the methods can be used with liquid concentrate. For powdered formula, some manufacturers recommend only the aseptic and single-bottle methods.

For ready-to-feed formula, sterilize the equipment according to the aseptic method; put the nipples, rings, and caps on the bottles; and store the bottles for up to 48 hours. Just before each feeding, clean the can top with hot soapy water, rinse the can, open it with a clean punch-type can opener, and pour the already sterile formula into the sterile bottle.

"**W**hen making up formula, don't get it close, GET IT RIGHT."—Ellyn Satter, *Child of Mine: Feeding with Love and Good Sense* (see The Parenting Bookshelf, page 143)

Sterilize Formula

THE ASEPTIC METHOD
(FOR LIQUID CONCENTRATE AND POWDER)

1. Wash the bottles, nipples, caps, rings, punch-type can opener (for liquid formula), and measuring scoop in hot, soapy water.

2. Put all of the clean equipment into a sterilizer or a large pan with a rack or towel on the bottom.

3. Cover the equipment with water, cover the pan, and bring the water to a boil. Boil for 5 minutes. Leave the equipment in the covered pan until the equipment is cool enough to handle.

4. In a kettle, bring fresh water just to a boil. Let it cool.

5. Wash and dry your hands, and then remove the equipment with tongs and place on a clean towel. Be careful not to touch the insides of the bottles or nipples.

6. Wash the top of the formula can with hot, soapy water, and rinse. If you're using liquid concentrate, shake the can well, and open it with the sterilized can opener.

7. Pour the directed amount of boiled water into the bottles. Add the formula. With the tongs, place the nipples upside down onto the bottles. Add the ring and cap, and tighten.

8. Shake the bottles. Store them in the refrigerator, and use them within 24 to 48 hours, as directed by the formula manufacturer.

HOW TO STERILIZE FORMULA, continued

THE TERMINAL STERILIZATION METHOD
(FOR LIQUID CONCENTRATE AND MOST BRANDS OF POWDER)

1. Wash the bottles, nipples, caps, rings, punch-type can opener (for liquid formula), and measuring scoop and a pitcher for mixing the formula in hot, soapy water.

2. Wash the top of the formula can with hot, soapy water, and rinse. If you're using liquid concentrate, shake the can well, and open it with the clean can opener.

3. Mix enough formula and cold water for a full day's use, stirring well.

4. Pour the prepared formula into the clean bottles. Place the nipples upside down on the bottles, and loosely put on the rings and caps.

5. Place the bottles in a sterilizer or on a rack or towel in a large pan with 3 inches of water. Cover the pan, and bring the water to a boil. Boil for 25 minutes. Turn off the heat, and leave the bottles in the covered pan for about an hour, until they are cool enough to touch.

6. Tighten the rings, and store the bottles in the refrigerator. Use them within 24 to 48 hours, as directed by the formula manufacturer.

SINGLE-BOTTLE METHOD I
(FOR LIQUID CONCENTRATE AND POWDER)

1. Wash the bottles, nipples, caps, rings, punch-type can opener (for liquid formula), and measuring scoop in hot, soapy water.

2. Put the directed amount of cold water into each bottle.

3. Place the nipples upside down on the bottles, and loosely put on the rings and caps.

4. Place the bottles in a sterilizer or on a rack or towel in a large pan. Pour in enough water to reach the level of the water in the bottles.

5. Cover the pan, and bring the water to a boil. Boil for 25 minutes. Turn off the heat, and leave the bottles in the covered pan for about an hour, until they are cool enough to touch.

6. Tighten the caps, and store the bottles at room temperature for as long as 48 hours.

7. Just before each feeding, wash the top of the formula can with hot, soapy water, and rinse. If you're using liquid concentrate, shake the can well, and open it with the clean can opener. Add the specified amount of formula to the bottle, and shake well. Feed the baby promptly.

SINGLE-BOTTLE METHOD II

1. Wash the bottles, nipples, caps, and rings in hot, soapy water.

HOW TO STERILIZE FORMULA, continued

2. Put the equipment into a sterilizer or on a rack or towel in a large pan. Cover everything with water, and bring the water to a boil. Boil for 5 minutes. Turn off the heat, and leave the bottles in the covered pan for about an hour, until they are cool enough to touch.

3. Wash and dry your hands, and then remove the equipment with tongs and place on a clean towel. Be careful not to touch the insides of the bottles or nipples.

4. Assemble the bottles, nipples, rings, and caps. Store them at room temperature for up to 48 hours.

5. At feeding time, bring fresh water just to a boil. Let it cool.

6. Wash the top of the formula can with hot, soapy water, and rinse. Open the can with a clean punch-type can opener. Add the measured formula and sterile water to the sterile bottles. Shake well, and feed the baby.

When your baby is about four months old, you can stop sterilizing formula and bottles. You must be sure, though, that the bottles are really clean. Before washing feeding equipment by hand, clean your sink and bottle brush. You can use a dishwasher instead if its water temperature reaches 140°F (as it probably does if the dishwasher has a heating element). Use the full cycle, including prerinse. Mix the formula in the bottle just before each feeding.

Even when you stop sterilizing bottles, it's a good idea to continue sterilizing nipples. Store them in a clean, dry, covered container.

CHECK YOUR
WATER SUPPLY

. . . .

Municipal water providers are required to monitor the safety of their water supplies, and most of these supplies are considered safe. Some, however, have high levels of contaminants that may be dangerous to infants, even after sterilization. You might check with your water department to find out whether local levels of bacteria, heavy metals, sodium, and nitrates are safe for a baby before deciding to use your tap water for mixing with formula. If you have a private well, have the water tested.

Municipal water supplies are chlorinated to lessen bacterial contamination, and sterilization kills most bacteria that survive chlorination. Chlorine itself may be dangerous in municipal water supplies, however; research has shown that it may be a cause of bladder cancer.

High nitrate levels, most common in farming areas, can react with a baby's hemoglobin to produce an anemic condition commonly known as "blue baby" (methemoglobinemia). Nitrate levels are *increased* by boiling the water.

Twenty percent of American homes may have tap water with high lead levels (15 micrograms or more per liter). Babies have been poisoned by lead in water used to mix formula. Lead can seriously damage the brain, nervous system, kidneys, and red blood cells, and this damage can permanently lower a child's IQ. For essential information on lead in water, see page 123.

Sodium in tap water can worsen dehydration when a baby is sick. High sodium levels can occur in coastal areas if seawater comes in contact with drinking-water supplies. Sodium contamination is also caused by home water softeners, although in many newer models the cold water bypasses the softening process. The Environmental Protection Agency has set 20 milligrams per liter as the maximum safe level for sodium in tap water.

Bottled water isn't necessarily purer or safer for your baby than tap water. The bottled-water industry is subject to the same standards as municipal water departments. Spring water and water labeled "drinking" or "filtered" can vary quite a lot in quality and probably isn't ideal for infants. (One baby-food company is now marketing "spring water with fluoride," an expensive and unnecessary product.) For contaminant-free water, choose bottles labeled "distilled," "demineralized," "de-ionized," or "purified."

A properly maintained home reverse-osmosis system also provides water free of contaminants. While you're investigating the safety of your water, check its fluoride content. Fluoride helps prevent cavities, so most doctors recommend fluoride supplements starting in infancy. But too much fluoride can cause spotting of a baby's teeth. If you plan to use tap water for mixing formula, and if the water contains fluoride in the proportion of 0.3 parts per million or more, don't give your baby fluoride supplements. If your water contains less fluoride, or if you are using only ready-to-feed formula or concentrated formula mixed with unfluoridated bottled water, your baby will need 0.25 milligrams of supplemental fluoride per day.

LEARN TO STORE AND WARM FORMULA SAFELY

. . . .

A can of formula can be safely stored, unopened, at room temperature until the expiration date on the can has passed. Once the can has been opened, liquid concentrate or ready-to-feed formula can be stored, tightly covered, in the refrigerator for up to 48 hours. Powdered formula can be stored, covered, in a cool, dry place for as long as the manufacturer recommends—typically four weeks for cow's-milk formula, three weeks for soy.

Prepared formula and open cans of liquid concentrate should be refrigerated at 35° to 40°F, because higher temperatures allow rapid bacterial growth. Measure your refrigerator temperature with an accurate thermometer; if the temperature is higher than 40°F, turn the thermostat down. If you must store prepared formula at higher than 40°F, throw it out after two hours. A bottle with formula left in it after a feeding can safely stay at room temperature for up to an hour. If the baby hasn't finished the formula in that time, throw it out.

Warming bottles isn't necessary. If you decide to warm them, though, do it just before each feeding, by holding the bottle under warm running tap water. Shake the bottle gently to distribute the warmth, and then test a drop or two on your wrist. Never warm a bottle by letting it sit out at room temperature or by heating it in a microwave. It's too easy to overheat formula in a microwave, and microwaving may destroy some vitamins.

When you are out with your baby for short periods, you can use bottles that have been prepared at home, chilled well, and kept unrefrigerated for no longer than two hours. When you are out for more than two hours, carry the bottles in a cooler. For even longer periods, you can bring along bottles sterilized with water in them, and mix in powdered formula just before each feeding (this is easiest if you measure out the powder at home and carry it in sterile disposable bags). Another option is to buy ready-to-feed bottles, but they are quite expensive.

KNOW HOW MUCH TO FEED

. . . .

Most babies can be trusted to take just as much formula as they need, as often as they need it. In the first couple of weeks, most want 3 to 6 ounces six to eight times a day, or 24 to 32 ounces per day. For a more precise guideline, figure that your baby needs 2.5 ounces per day for each pound of the baby's weight. This will hold true until the baby reaches 12 to 13 pounds, at which point his intake will stabilize at about 32 ounces per day.

The exact amount of formula your baby takes each day will depend on his age, growth pattern, activity level, and factors such as illness and other discomforts. If you're worried about your baby's growth, your baby's doctor or nurse can show you how it is progressing on a growth chart.

Some babies overfeed, to the point of obesity. Within an hour or two after a feeding, a baby may act hungry again, and take several more ounces of formula. Or he may space his feedings more widely, but consume tremendous amounts at each. A baby who seems to overconsume—especially if he also has intestinal symptoms, such as spitting up, passing a lot of gas, an irritated rectal area, or frequent runny stools—may be sensitive to something in the formula, in which case a change should be considered. It may also be that the baby needs extra sucking. A pacifier or bottle of water might satisfy the baby and keep him from overconsuming formula.

PLAN TO BOTTLE-FEED LIKE A BREASTFEEDER

According to some studies, breastfed children tend to score higher on IQ tests than those who are bottle-fed (see page 28), and this may originate, in part, from their frequent and prolonged contact with their mothers. When a woman breastfeeds, her face, voice, and touch are always present during feedings, stimulating her baby to look at her, "talk" to her, touch her, and play with her. Bottle-feeding, though never so physically intimate, can still be an opportunity for parent-child social interaction. Too often, parents ignore this opportunity. Because holding a baby for bottle-feeding requires the use of two arms, it quickly becomes an unpleasant chore for many parents. So they lay the baby down and, in one way or another, prop the bottle up. Bottle propping is dangerous: It can make a young baby choke.

When a bottle-fed baby reaches about three months of age, he may be expected to feed himself. Although some parents see self-feeding as a developmental accomplishment, it deprives a baby of some very important contact and stimulation. Imagine what a baby misses out on when he spends his day sitting in an infant seat, feeding himself.

The bottle can become unhealthful in other ways, too. Babies often drop bottles and then put them back into their mouths— along with dirt and bacteria from the floor or the ground. Older babies and toddlers who carry around bottles all day, or go to sleep sucking on them, risk serious tooth decay.

Plan to bottle-feed as if you're breastfeeding. Tell yourself that the bottle belongs to you, not your child. Hold your baby in your arms whenever you feed him, and have your partner and other care-givers do the same thing. Let him control his feeding as a breast-fed baby does: Wait for him to open his mouth rather than pushing the nipple in yourself. Be patient when he pauses in sucking; don't stimulate him to suck continuously. Even if there is formula left in the bottle, let your baby stop drinking when he signals that he has had enough. Just as most breastfed babies drift off to sleep in Mom's arms, let your bottle-fed baby do the same, rather than putting him into his crib wide awake.

PURCHASES TO CONSIDER

Before your baby is born, you might buy two weeks' worth of formula, in ready-to-feed or liquid concentrate form. Before you buy more, you'll want to be sure your baby tolerates the type of formula you've chosen. Figure you'll need 18 to 24 ounces of prepared formula per day for these first two weeks. Start with cow's-milk formula unless the baby's doctor has advised you to do otherwise. When buying formula, always check the expiration date, since sometimes stores carry outdated formula. After the initial formula purchase, you can save money by buying formula in a large quantity from a big-box store. You might also save by using a generic brand.

Choosing bottles can be a bit overwhelming, because there are many different types. The best are easy to clean and have accurate measuring indicators. Angled ones are supposed to make it easier to keep the nipple filled, but this is just as easy with straight bottles. Bottles molded into unusual shapes or split down the middle for self-feeding are nearly impossible to keep clean.

Bottles are made from various plastics and from glass. Glass bottles are easiest to clean but are heavier than plastic and harder to find. Glass is also easy to sterilize and most accurate for measuring.

Some bottles come with disposable liners, which are supposed to cause less air swallowing. They don't. The disposable bags can lessen the work of sterilization somewhat, because they are sterile from the start. But you can't sterilize formula in the bags; the bags would break. And you can't use the bag to measure formula concentrate or water, as you can a bottle. Instead, you have to mix the formula in a sterile container before pouring it into the bags. You can avoid this step by buying ready-to-feed formula, but in any case you'll need to boil the nipples and caps. In the end, the extra cost of a "feeding system" that uses disposable bags probably outweighs the benefits.

Most bottles come in either of two sizes, 4 ounces and 8 ounces. Four-ounce bottles make more sense for babies who are taking only 2 to 4 ounces at a feeding. You can buy 8-ounce bottles later, when your baby is drinking 5 to 6 ounces at a feeding.

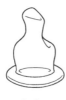

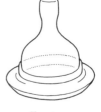

Standard   *Orthodontic*   *Flat-top*   *European*

THINGS TO GET

For Bottle-Feeding

- Two weeks' worth of formula
- A baby-bottle sterilizer or large covered pan
- Bottle and nipple brushes (separate or combined)
- A 32-ounce glass measuring cup for measuring water and liquid formula
- Tongs for lifting sterilized bottles
- A long-handled stainless-steel spoon for mixing formula
- A bottle drying rack and a bottle organizer (for storage)

Nipples come in various shapes and flow speeds. Your choice of nipples will be limited somewhat by your choice of bottles. If possible, try a few different nipples; your baby may do better with one type than another. The basic shapes are standard, orthodontic, flat-top, and European.

- *Standard nipples,* which fit most regular bottles (that is, bottles not made for disposable liners), are short with a narrow base.
- *Orthodontic nipples* have a wide base and a top supposedly shaped like the nipple of a breast when it is flattened in a baby's mouth. These nipples must be positioned with the hole at the top of the baby's mouth.
- *Flat-top nipples* come with the Playtex "nurser," a bottle used with disposable liners. These wide-based nipples extend into the baby's mouth when he sucks.

◆ *European nipples* are longer, with a wide base. They fit only the wide-mouth bottles made by Avent.

Nipples are made of latex rubber or silicone. Silicone nipples are definitely preferable. Rubber has a taste and odor and deteriorates faster than silicone does. Rubber is also harder to clean and so should be washed by hand, not in a dishwasher.

Don't bother buying a bottle warmer; these generally take too long to heat. Besides, most babies will take cold or room-temperature formula.

CHAPTER 5

The Nursery, and Whether You Need One

Dreaming about the perfect nursery—with wallpaper, a fancy crib, and a rocking chair—is a happy indulgence during pregnancy. For many expectant parents, buying furniture, painting, and setting up the baby's room is a rite of passage that can't be skipped.

The fact of the matter is, though, that the typical baby spends little time in her nursery. In the early months, it is usually easier for the parents to keep the baby close by at night, in a bassinet or even in their own bed.

If you have the space and budget for a designer nursery, enjoy making the fantasy a reality. But don't feel obligated to spend a lot of money. Grandparents may delight in buying a crib, dresser, or rocker. You can do fine with some borrowed items. If space is an issue or if you prefer to have the baby close at hand, you might set up a dresser in your bedroom and wait until after the baby is born to decide whether or when she needs her own room. Instead of decorating a nursery, you might put your nesting urge into creating one or two nursing areas, each with a comfortable armchair and a small table on which you can set a drink and a telephone.

SLEEPING ARRANGEMENTS

Although mothers and babies have slept together at least as long as mammals have roamed the Earth, warnings about the dangers of bed-sharing are worrying new parents. In 1999, the Consumer Product Safety Commission recommended against parents and babies sleeping together, although many parents, physicians, and scientists—including one of the commissioners—disagreed.

Since then, the American Academy of Pediatrics has recommended that nursing mothers, at least, sleep close to their babies. There are good reasons for this:

◆ Moms and dads who sleep with their babies say that they enjoy the closeness and find it makes nighttime parenting easier.

◆ Being close to the baby during the night means being more aware of her cues and therefore more responsive to her needs. Babies who sleep with their parents cry less than babies who sleep alone.

◆ Because bed-sharing mothers nurse frequently, they produce more milk than they would if their babies slept in another room. This can be especially important for women who must spend time apart from their babies during the day.

◆ Bed-sharing may reduce a baby's risk of succumbing to Sudden Infant Death Syndrome (SIDS). Dr. James McKenna, an expert on infant sleep, believes that when a parent and baby are close enough during nighttime sleep to sense each other in at least two of four ways—sight, scent, sound, and touch—the baby is much less likely to experience prolonged sleep apnea, which causes SIDS. The adult's close breathing, McKenna thinks, may help regulate a baby's own breathing.

You may worry that you won't get much sleep with a baby in your bed. Studies have found that bed-sharing mothers and babies wake more often, but they go back to sleep sooner and so get more sleep overall than mothers and babies who sleep separately. Since the baby sleeping with her parents scarcely needs to whimper to get a meal, she may never wake Dad with her cries.

You may fear that sleeping with your baby will make her too dependent. But researchers have found that babies who sleep with their parents develop into children who are independent, sociable, confident, and able to handle stress well. Children who have always slept alone, say the researchers, are judged by their parents as more dependent, harder to control, less happy, more fearful, and more prone to tantrums.

There are hazards to avoid in bed-sharing, but there are hazards in laying the baby to sleep anywhere. Wherever the baby sleeps, the dangers are mostly the same: pillows, toys, and quilts that could suffocate; cords and ties that could strangle; gaps in which a baby could become wedged; heights from which she could fall; and overheating, which increases the risk of SIDS. Bed-sharing poses the additional risk of overlying, but this is extremely unlikely to happen unless other children are sharing the bed or a parent is intoxicated or utterly exhausted. Generally, adults have a sense of their own boundaries even while asleep; this is why you don't fall out of bed at night. Besides following the "Guidelines for Safe Baby Sleep," bed-sharing parents will want to put a waterproof pad on their mattress, to protect it from milk, spit-up, and leaky diapers.

Safe Baby Sleep

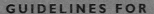

- Use a firm mattress that fits the bed or crib frame well, without gaps in which a baby could possibly become wedged.

- Stretch the sheet tightly around the mattress.

- Avoid nightclothes with strings or ties, both for the baby and, if you're sharing the bed, for yourself and your partner.

- Keep the baby's face uncovered.

- Leave off the bed pillows, comforters, feather beds, stuffed animals, lambskins, beanbags, and other soft things that could pose a risk of suffocation.

- Put the baby on her back to sleep. Babies sleeping on their backs are less likely to succumb to SIDS.

- Don't smoke, and don't let other people smoke in your home. Exposure to tobacco, both during pregnancy and during infancy, is associated with a higher risk of SIDS.

- Avoid overheating the room in which the baby sleeps, and avoid overdressing the baby.

- Don't lay the baby to sleep near dangling cords or sashes.

- Don't leave a young baby, especially one born prematurely, to sleep in a car seat or infant seat. If the baby's upper body is inadequately supported, her airway may become blocked.

IF YOUR BABY SLEEPS IN A CRIB:

- Make sure the rails are spaced no wider than 2⅜ inches apart.

- If you use a crib bumper, make sure it has at least six ties, each no longer than 9 inches.
- Hang any crib mobile well out of the baby's reach, and remove it when the baby starts to sit or reaches five months of age, whichever comes first.
- When the baby starts to sit, lower the mattress so that she can't fall out or climb over the side rail.
- When she learns to stand, set the mattress at its lowest level and remove anything she could stand on.
- When she reaches a height of 32 inches or the side rail reaches less than three-quarters of her height, move her to another bed.
- Remove any crib gym when a baby can get up on all fours.
- If your house is cool at night, dress the baby in a blanket sleeper instead of using a blanket. If you do use a blanket, make sure the baby's head remains uncovered.

IF YOUR BABY SLEEPS WITH YOU:

- Don't share a waterbed with your baby, because the surface could hamper breathing if your baby were to turn face down.
- Don't sleep with the baby on a sofa or an overstuffed chair.
- If your bed has head- or footboard railings, make sure they are spaced no wider than 2⅜ inches apart.
- Don't use bed rails in the baby's first year, because she could become wedged between the mattress and the side rail.

SAFE BABY SLEEP, continued

◆ Don't place the bed against the wall or against other furniture, because the baby could become trapped in between.

◆ Don't leave the baby to sleep alone in your bed.

◆ Fasten back your hair, if it is very long.

◆ Any time you've had a lot to drink, taken drugs that may cause you to sleep soundly, or become extremely exhausted, put the baby to sleep in a separate bed.

◆ Don't let an older sibling share a bed with a baby less than a year old.

Adapted from a list prepared by Patricia Donohue-Carey for the September-October 2002 issue of Mothering

For most of the benefits of bed-sharing with no risk of over-lying, you have several options. You might put your baby to sleep in a cradle or bassinet close to your own bed. You might buy a bedside sleeper, a baby bed that securely attaches to an adult bed; with one of these, your baby will sleep on a separate surface, but you will still be able to reach her without getting up (see page 58). Or you might try a Snuggle Nest, a padded plastic baby bed designed to fit between the pillows of the parents' bed. Intended to prevent any possibility of a baby's rolling over, overheating, or suffocating, the Snuggle Nest is outgrown at about three months. For ordering information, see Other Resources for New Parents, page 146.

BABY BEDS

Even if you have decided that your baby will sleep with you, you'll probably want to get her some sort of bed of her own. You'll use it when she is sleeping but you and your partner are up, or when you and your partner simply want the bed to yourselves for a while.

Today, most people consider cribs to be essential baby furniture, but they really aren't. For the early months you may prefer a cradle, a bassinet, or a baby bed that attaches to your bed. For a longer period, you might get by with a play yard.

Cradles

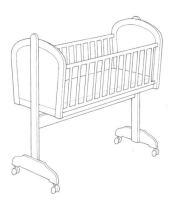

These old-fashioned baby beds, with their lovely rocking motion, are so well loved that many families pass them from one generation to the next. In my tight-knit obstetrical unit, the staff passed the same cradle from nurse to nurse as our families expanded.

If you are offered an old cradle, make sure it is sturdy and safe to use. If the sides have slats, they should be no farther than 2⅜ inches apart. The mattress should be in good condition and should fit snugly in the cradle. If you need a new mattress, have one made, or make your own with 1- to 2-inch-thick high-density foam.

Similar to a cradle is a new product from Australia, the Amby Baby Hammock Motion Swing. This is essentially a sling suspended from a spring that hangs from a metal frame. The baby sleeps on her back, swaddled in the sling. When she moves, the sling bounces gently to help her get back to sleep. A baby can sleep until the age of nine to twelve months in the Amby. For ordering information, see Other Resources for New Parents, page 146.

Bassinets

Like cradles, these long-legged baskets work well in the early months of a baby's life. Some bassinets rock, and most have wheels on which they can be moved from room to room. Many modern bassinets are made of sturdy wood rather than woven fiber.

You may prefer to borrow rather than buy a bassinet, because you'll use it for such a short time. If you decide to buy one secondhand, pass up any made before the mid-1970s; they may be coated with lead-based paint. Besides, old bassinets are often weak and unstable. If a used bassinet has folding legs, make sure that strong, secure locks will keep them extended during use. Make sure the mattress is in good condition and fits snugly, with no more than two fingers' space between it and the side of the bassinet. If the mattress is inadequate, you can buy a replacement at a store that sells baby furnishings. Get a mattress pad, too. A pillowcase may work well as a sheet.

If you are considering buying both a bassinet and a play yard, you may save money by buying one of the bassinet add-ons that are available for most play yards (see opposite).

Bedside Sleepers

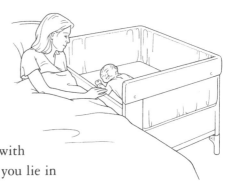

For parents who want to avoid getting up for night feedings but don't want the baby in their bed, this is the best option. About the size of a portable crib, a bedside sleeper has straps that keep it tightly attached and level with your mattress, so that when you lie in bed the baby is just several inches away. These beds are expensive, and they are outgrown as fast as a cradle or bassinet. If a friend has a used one, you might ask whether you could borrow it.

Portable Cribs

These are also referred to as miniature cribs and Grandma cribs. Made of wood or metal, these small cribs can be moved around the house, because they fit easily through doorways. Although a portable crib uses regular crib mattresses and bedding, the crib is usable for only four to six months; it is no longer safe when the baby can push herself up on all fours. For an occasional baby bed that will serve you longer, consider getting a play yard.

Play Yards

These modern versions of the old-fashioned wooden playpen, made of aluminum tubing and mesh sides, weigh about 20 to 25 pounds and fold up for travel. With or without an optional bassinet, which

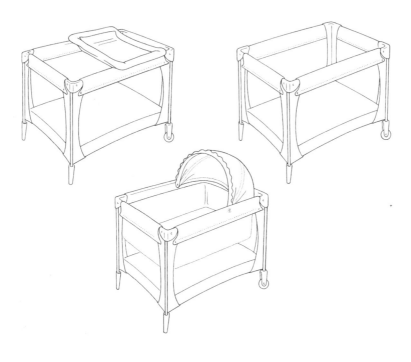

is suspended from the top rail, a play yard can take the place of a crib when you are traveling with the baby or she is napping at home.

Many manufacturers have recalled their play yard models because of dangerous defects. If you buy or borrow a used play yard, be sure to call the manufacturer to ask about any recall. You'll also want to buy a new mattress and fitted sheets for the play yard, bassinet, or both.

Cribs

These come in a variety of styles. The best have a side that can be dropped easily and quietly with one hand, and two mattress height options. If you are looking at a crib without a drop side, make sure you are tall enough to be able to reach down and lift the baby comfortably. A second drop side and more mattress height options are unnecessary and generally make the crib more expensive.

Some cribs can be converted into low beds for toddlers, but this feature makes a crib more expensive. Besides, if you have another baby in a couple of years you'll probably want to continue using the crib as a crib. Your toddler can just as easily move into a twin-size bed.

Some cribs come with under-bed storage. Unfortunately, the drawers in these cribs tend to be poorly constructed. A dresser is more useful, if you have room for it.

Crib mishaps are one of the leading causes of injury to infants and toddlers. All new cribs meet government safety standards, but older ones may not. If you are considering borrowing a crib, make sure it is no more than a few years old. Cribs manufactured before 1979 may have slats that are more widely spaced than the currently recommended maximum (2⅜ inches), and cribs made before 1974 may be covered with lead-based paint. Older cribs may be worn and rickety, too.

One of the most common causes of crib injuries is a baby or toddler's attempt to climb out. To avoid falls:

◆ Lower the mattress as far as possible as soon as the baby can sit up.

◆ When the baby can stand, make sure there is nothing in the crib that she can stand on.

◆ Especially when your baby becomes a toddler, be sure not to place the crib next to any furniture that she could use as a step to climb out.

◆ Move your child out of the crib when she is 32 inches tall or when the side rail reaches less than three-quarters of her height.

CRIB MATTRESSES. New cribs usually don't come with mattresses. Used cribs usually do, but it is generally recommended that parents buy a new mattress for a used crib, because new fire-resistance standards for crib mattresses were put in place in 2004. Also, studies in Great Britain and New Zealand suggest a higher risk of SIDS when mattresses are reused. The theory is that mold or mildew combines with the fireproofing chemical in the mattress to produce a toxic gas; the more a mattress has been used, the more likely it is that mold and mildew are present.

Crib mattresses come in two basic types, foam and innerspring. All crib mattresses made today, of either type, are hypoallergenic. The best ones are very firm. This doesn't necessarily mean you should buy an innerspring; even less expensive foam mattresses can be quite firm, whereas some innerspring mattresses are too soft.

To evaluate a foam mattress, press it in the center on both sides at the same time; the foam should compact little. In general, the heavier the mattress is, the denser the foam. But even dense foam mattresses weigh less than innerspring mattresses, and so are easier to handle when you change the sheet. To evaluate an innerspring mattress, don't worry about the number of coils. Again, test for firmness by pressing on the mattress.

Besides firmness, other features to consider in a crib mattress are the covering material, border rods, and ventilation holes. A thin vinyl covering with vinyl edging will deteriorate over time. Look for thick double or triple laminates and edges with fabric

BEFORE ACCEPTING A USED CRIB

Take These Precautions

◆ Look for a Consumer Product Safety Commission approval label; this indicates that the crib meets safety standards.

◆ Make sure the corner posts are no more than 1/16 inch higher than the end panel, so the baby's clothes can't catch on the posts.

◆ Make sure the panels don't have cutouts in which a baby's head could possibly become trapped.

◆ Shop for a new mattress.

◆ Set the mattress in its lowest position, and make sure its top surface is at least 26 inches from the top of the railing.

◆ Check the side-rail releases to make sure they can't be reached from inside the crib.

◆ Rub your hands over the wood and the hardware to make sure there are no sharp edges or splinters.

◆ Make sure that you have or can order the instructions that came with the crib.

binding. Border rods at the top and bottom edges provide extra support and durability. Ventilation holes help prevent mildew from developing and help keep the seams from splitting when the baby starts jumping.

CRIB BEDDING. Many parents choose decorations for an entire room—paint, wallpaper, rug, and so on—to match the bedding they have chosen for a crib, usually in a packaged set. But such bedding sets typically include fluffy comforters, which pose a suffocation hazard. It's best to buy the bedding pieces you need separately.

Unless your crib mattress is truly waterproof—that is, there are no tears in the covering material—the first things you'll need are a couple of waterproof sheets. These are machine-washable and -dryable sheets of rubber covered on both sides with cotton flannel. Buy flat ones instead of the more expensive fitted ones, because the mattress cover will keep the flat ones in place.

A quilted mattress pad goes over the waterproof sheet to make the bed cooler and a little softer. Avoid really puffy mattress pads, because they can increase a baby's risk of SIDS. Some pads come with rubber backing, and so might save you from having to buy waterproof sheets, but I've found that these pads can't be dried in the dryer without the backing disintegrating. Consider buying two mattress pads.

Fitted crib sheets are made in three varieties: combed cotton, thin flannel, and jersey knit. The flannel and jersey knit ones tend to be easier to put on the mattress. They are also much softer and warmer than combed cotton, and therefore less shocking for a baby laid on them. Sheets elasticized all the way around are much easier to put over the mattress. If your crib mattress is especially thick, make sure the sheets will cover it. Consider buying four crib sheets.

Meant to keep the baby from hurting her head against the crib slats, bumper pads are now frowned on because they are thought to pose a risk of smothering. If you use a crib bumper, make sure it is flat, thin, and filled with polyester rather than flammable cotton. The bumper should tie to the crib slats in at least six places, and the ties should be no longer than 9 inches each. You can make your own bumper pad using thin polyester batting. Remove the pad from the crib as soon as the baby can stand, or she might use it as a step to climb out of the crib.

Dust ruffles are pretty, but they serve no purpose besides hiding the crib hardware and items stored underneath.

Sleep positioners, designed to keep babies on their sides as they sleep, are no longer recommended, because babies are at the lowest risk of SIDS when they sleep on their backs.

CHANGING TABLES

With a lightweight flannel receiving blanket on which to lay the baby, any flat surface can be a changing table. My favorite was the bed. Other parents use the crib, the couch, or a rug on the floor. Most parents have more than one place in the home where they change the baby.

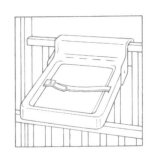

If you'd like an official changing station, you have many options. You could get a small changing station as an optional add-on to a play yard, or you could buy a changing table that attaches to the front of a crib and folds down when not in use. If space allows, you might

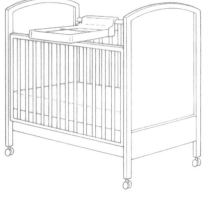

prefer a freestanding changing table, with shelves underneath where you can put things that the baby might otherwise kick or toss to the floor. But any of these items will quickly outlive its usefulness. If you must have a changing table, you might want to borrow rather than buy one.

Baby dressers come with changing-table tops. But baby furniture is expensive; one of these dressers costs about $500 to $600. Any low dresser or table will serve just as well as a changing station. Just cover a foam pad with waterproof fabric and place it on top. With any elevated changing surface, of course, the baby should never be left alone.

DRESSERS

· ·

An ordinary chest of drawers is generally cheaper than a baby dresser and may last a child her whole life. Try to find one that is sturdy, with drawers that open and close easily. Drawers with roller bearings on the sides are easier to use than those with tracks on the bottom, but tracks on the bottom are better than no tracks at all. High-quality dressers are dovetailed; that is, the sides are interlocked with the front and the back rather than just butted and glued. A laminated top will resist staining and scratching.

If you lack the money or space for a dresser, consider closet organizers. These mix-and-match systems can provide drawers, shelves, and cubbies. You can either install the components yourself or get help from a professional.

ROCKERS AND OTHER CHAIRS

· ·

No dream nursery would be complete without a rocking chair. An old-fashioned rocking chair may work well for you, if it moves smoothly and quietly. For the most comfort, you'll probably want a padded seat. Actually, though, the chair might get more use in your bedroom or even the living room. And you might like the chair more if it's not a rocker.

Today, gliders are more popular than rocking chairs. Gliders take up less space, they are generally more comfortable, and they provide rhythmic motion with less effort. Some come with a reclining feature and a locking mechanism to keep toddlers from pinching their fingers in the gliding track. A new glider costs about $350 without an ottoman, which you probably don't need.

Although sometimes helpful in calming a fussy baby, a rocker or glider isn't a necessity for new parents. Any supportive armchair may be comfortable for nursing or soothing your baby.

OTHER FURNISHINGS

Electronic Baby Monitors

If you work in the kitchen, office, or somewhere else distant from where the baby is napping, one of these devices may allow you to hear her cries. A baby monitor is of little use, however, to most families who live in small houses and apartments.

Because baby monitors operate on the same channels as portable phones, your monitor may pick up your neighbors' phone conversations, and your neighbors may be able to hear your conversations in the nursery or bedroom. This could happen quite frequently if you live in an urban area or if your cordless phone and baby monitor are on the same frequency. For the sake of privacy, you'll want to keep the monitor turned off when you don't need it.

Soft Lighting

For nighttime diaper changes, you'll want a lamp with a low-wattage bulb—15 to 25 watts—or a dimmer switch for the overhead lamp. Many parents use plug-in night-lights, but these can be hazardous unless the outlet is out of reach of a crawling baby and away from flammable materials such as bedding and drapes.

Other Items

Many parents find that a regular bed is the most useful item in a nursery. It's perfect for nighttime nursings, diaper changing, playing, and lying down together before putting baby to sleep.

You may also want a laundry hamper and trash basket, a diaper pail (see page 73), and a CD player or radio. Finally, you might securely fasten a mobile over the crib or changing table.

CHAPTER 6

Dressing and Grooming Your Baby

Most parents assemble necessities for the newborn a few weeks before the due date, so they know that all the baby's things will be available, washed, and organized in time for his arrival. You may want to put off shopping, though, until after you sort through any baby-shower gifts and hand-me-downs sent your way. Then you can make a list of only the things you need. To help you make your choices, you might bring along to the store a friend or relative who has had children. Buy what you can afford, and have fun doing it!

THE LAYETTE

. . . .

What *is* a layette? This old-fashioned term, French for "small box" or "small drawer," refers to the clothing and accessories, such as towels and blankets, intended to meet a newborn's initial needs.

Baby clothes are sized according to age: newborn, 3 months, 6 months, 9 months, and 12 months. Some are sized according to a range, such as 6 to 12 months. Since newborns grow so quickly, you may want to buy just a few pieces of very small clothing, and even these might be 3- or 6-month size rather than newborn size. You can always buy more when you learn what styles you prefer. If you're going to have a baby shower, of course, you'll probably want to delay buying any clothing until afterward. How much clothing you ultimately need will depend partially on how often you do laundry.

If you want to follow the old rule of pink for girls and blue for boys but you don't yet know your baby's sex, you might put a deposit on two sets of layette items at a children's store. After the baby is born, you can bring home the set of your choice.

The most practical baby clothes are cotton knits with snaps or zippers down the front and legs to make diaper changes easy. Cotton is soft and breathable, and stretch knits are generally easiest to put on and take off and comfortable for the baby. Snaps and zippers are easier to fasten and unfasten than buttons, which pose a choking hazard if they come loose. Make sure that snaps are securely attached and that they don't come apart too easily. Avoid clothes that fasten down the back, since the fasteners could be irritating to a baby who spends most of his time on his back, and it's a bother to have to flip a baby over to fasten or unfasten snaps.

You'll need to decide whether you want to buy flame-retardant sleepwear, which stops burning as soon as it is withdrawn from any flames. For some years, federal law forbid the sale of non-flame-retardant nightclothes, but in 1998 the Consumer Product Safety Commission retracted this rule, because only loose-fitting clothing, such as long gowns, substantially increases the risk of

THINGS TO GET FOR

Your Baby's Layette

THREE TO SIX RECEIVING BLANKETS. These are thin cotton blankets for swaddling, extra warmth, and privacy when Mom is nursing in public. The most popular kind are made of cotton waffle-weave fabric, which is cool in summer and warm in winter. Others are made of jersey knit or cotton flannel. You can make your own receiving blankets by cutting 36- to 45-inch square pieces of fabric and stitching a rolled hem on all sides.

ONE OR TWO HOODED TOWELS. There is no reason you can't use an ordinary bath towel, but baby towels have a fine, soft weave, and the hood makes it easy to keep the baby's head warm.

TWO TO FOUR WASHCLOTHS. Again, you can use ordinary washcloths, but those made for babies are softer.

THREE TO SIX UNDERSHIRTS. These are better to use than body suits before the umbilical cord falls off. If you're squeamish about pulling a shirt over the baby's head, get the kind that has snaps or ties on the front.

FOUR TO EIGHT BODY SUITS (such as Onesies). Long pullover undershirts that snap at the baby's crotch, these

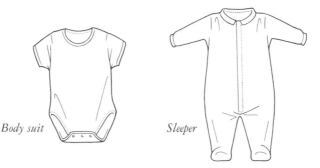

Body suit   *Sleeper*

YOUR BABY'S LAYETTE, continued

don't ride up the way ordinary undershirts do. Short-sleeved body suits can be worn on their own in hot weather.

FOUR TO EIGHT LIGHTWEIGHT SLEEPERS ("STRETCHIES"). In the early weeks, your baby may wear these day and night. Size 3 to 6 months should fit fine.

TWO TO FOUR ROMPERS (COVERALLS). These are like sleepers but without feet. Available in various fabrics and styles, rompers are good for outings. Pick short-sleeved ones for warm weather and long-sleeved ones for colder months. For easy diaper changes, rompers should snap all the way down both legs.

TWO TO FOUR INFANT GOWNS (KIMONOS). Long nightgowns with elastic at the bottom make diaper changes easy. Avoid the ones with string instead of elastic, because the string could be a strangulation hazard.

TWO TO FOUR BLANKET SLEEPERS. Intended for cold nights, these heavy sleepers come either with a sack-like lower end or with legs. Blanket sleepers eliminate the need for blankets in the bassinet or crib.

ONE OR TWO SWEATERS. Choose cotton for summer, warmer fabrics for winter.

THREE TO SIX PAIRS OF SOCKS OR BOOTIES. You won't lose them as fast if they fit snugly. Booties should be soft; babies who are not walking yet have no need for shoes.

TWO TO FOUR HATS. You'll need one or two newborn caps of lightweight cotton knit, and one or two hats for outdoors. Choose a wide-brimmed cotton hat for the warm-weather months, and heavy cotton, acrylic, or polar fleece that covers the ears for cold-weather months.

ONE SNOWSUIT OR BUNTING, if your winters are cold. One-piece insulated suits with arms and legs, snowsuits can be hard to get on and off. Sack-like buntings are easier to use, but even those with divided legs shouldn't be used in car seats, because they keep the belts from being pulled snugly. Instead, strap the baby into the car seat, put a blanket on top, and tuck it in well behind the baby. The best buntings are made from soft fleece or another breathable fabric rather than waterproof nylon.

burns. Besides, several studies have linked chemical flame retardants with cancer. Synthetics such as polyester are naturally flame-retardant; they melt, but they don't burn. Flame-retardant cotton is chemically treated and expensive. If you prefer to dress your baby in untreated cotton, just make sure it fits snugly.

Before the birth, wash all of the baby's clothes. This will soften them and remove dust, excess dye, and other potential allergens. Some of the clothes may shrink, in which case you'll be able to use them sooner than you thought.

The best detergents for a baby's laundry are those labeled hypoallergenic. Don't use fabric softeners or dryer sheets, which can leave a flammable residue on flame-retardant garments. On any clothes, the residue has an irritating smell and may cause nasal stuffiness. Special stain removers are marketed for baby clothes, but most stains come out if the clothing is immediately placed in cold water.

DIAPERS AND
DIAPERING

. . . .

You and your partner can plan on changing about 2,800 diapers a year for about three years.

You'll need to decide whether to start with cloth diapers or disposables. Today, 95 percent of parents choose disposables, for their convenience. They are expensive, though—about $800 per year. Whether you are more concerned about this cost or about the cost to the environment, you may prefer cloth diapers. Many parents who choose cloth say they prefer having natural, breathable cotton against their babies' skin.

Some parents relieve their worry about the environment by buying organic disposables. Most of these are chemical-free and contain unbleached cotton for absorbency in place of a gel pad. Organic brands include Tushies, Bambo, Moltex, Nature Boy, and Nature Girl. Only the last two are fully biodegradable.

Parents who choose cloth can either use a diaper service, if one is available, or wash their own diapers. Using a diaper service can be as expensive as using disposables. The most environmentally responsible, least expensive way to go is to launder cloth diapers at home.

The diaper question isn't really the either/or sort. Parents who use cloth diapers often use disposables for travel, nights, or both. Disposables can save parents repeated nighttime rousings or frequent sheet changes.

Disposable Diapers

These come in three styles: basic, ultrathin, and premium (or "supreme"). Today, all disposables except the organic ones come with a polymer gel filling that absorbs the baby's urine, so the baby's bottom really does stay dry. Basic diapers are bulkiest but cost the least. Ultrathins are less bulky and more absorbent; they can hold up to 16 ounces of urine. Premiums, which cost about 25 percent more than other disposables, have a soft outer layer that feels like cloth instead of like a plastic bag and Velcro-type closures instead of tape. *Consumer Reports* finds that most disposable diapers, regardless of style or brand, generally fit well and don't leak.

In the early weeks, you will need about 100 diapers per week. You can buy either newborn-size disposables, which fit babies under 8 pounds and have a special cutout for airing the umbilical cord stump, or size 1 diapers, which most hospitals use. To protect the cord stump with size 1 diapers, turn down the top of the diaper to the outside.

It's easy to stock up on diapers when you do your grocery shopping, but be aware that disposables are cheaper at warehouse stores and other stores that sell diapers in large quantities. Some of these stores have their own brands of disposable diapers, which generally are cheapest of all.

You will want a lidded pail for containing used diapers. A foot-operated garbage pail works well; you might add a charcoal filter or a nontoxic deodorizer cake to reduce odor. Or you can buy a special pail such as the Diaper Genie, which seals each diaper in a scented plastic bag. These pails cost more, of course, and refilling the stock of disposable bags adds to the cost (although with some brands you can use standard plastic bags instead of the special scented ones). The lid of a diaper pail should be very difficult for a toddler to open.

Even if you decide to diaper only with disposables, you may want to buy a dozen cloth diapers. They are handy as spit-up cloths and useful for many other jobs.

Cloth Diapers

Despite their decline in popularity, cloth diapers come in an enormous variety of fabrics and styles.

DIAPER FABRICS. Most are cotton—usually gauze, bird's-eye, terry, or flannel. Some are cotton jersey, twill, fleece, or knit. There are even cotton velour diapers.

Cotton Diaper Fabrics

GAUZE. A soft, loosely woven, finely spun fabric that makes a comfortable, absorbent diaper with good air flow.

BIRD'S-EYE. A tightly woven, very absorbent fabric that lasts the longest and costs the most.

TERRY. Durable and more absorbent than any of the other diaper fabrics, but also more bulky.

FLANNEL. The most popular fabric for diapers. A soft, loose twill weave with a slightly napped surface.

Hemp is becoming increasingly popular for use in diapers because of its durability, absorbency, and natural antimicrobial properties. The coarse fiber comes from the inner bark of the hemp plant. The hemp used in the diapers now on the market is grown without chemical pesticides or fertilizers. The fiber is used to make French terry (terry cloth looped on only one side), fleece, and jersey fabric, all of which are used in fewer layers to make diapers just as absorbent as any made of cotton. Fewer layers means trimmer diapers and a shorter drying time. Because hemp is so absorbent, is has a reputation for stinking. Thorough washing is essential to remove odors.

Some diapers are made of synthetic fleece—Micro fleece, Polartec fleece, and WindPro fleece. All of these are highly breathable, lightweight, durable, stain-resistant, fast-drying, and very soft. They are not, however, absorbent. Heavier fleeces are used for diaper covers and some all-in-one diapers. Lightweight fleeces are used on the inside of some diapers, so the moisture passes through and the baby feels drier.

A cotton-polyester blend popular for diapers is Sherpa terry. This is the brushed, washed terry knit that is used for baby towels. It has a fluffy, very soft feel. Because the cotton content is high, the fabric is very absorbent as well.

DIAPER STYLES. Cloth diapers come in six styles: unfolded, prefolded, shaped, fitted, all-in-one, and pocket.

Unfolded diapers are large rectangles or squares of thin cotton (flannel, terry, or gauze) or hemp. Many parents prefer these, for various reasons: They cost less; they dry fast; and they are most versatile. You can fold them to fit the baby best, with the thickest part where the baby needs it most. The same diapers, folded in various ways, will fit a baby from birth through toddlerhood. You'll need pins or Snappi clips (which fasten with tiny claws) to hold these diapers in place.

Prefolds are the most popular style of cloth diaper. They are sewn with several layers down the center section, so little or no additional folding is needed. These diapers can be used without pins or other fasteners if you have diaper covers with Velco-type closures.

The best prefolds are diaper-service quality, or "DSQ." These are made of a very soft, absorbent cotton, which comes bleached or unbleached and may even be organically grown. Standard-ply DSQ prefolds are four layers thick on the sides and six layers thick in the middle. Premium DSQ prefolds are four layers thick on the sides and eight layers thick in the middle. The very best DSQ diapers are made in China; these are what most diaper services use. Some prefolds sold in stores and labeled "diaper-service quality" are really no such thing. To get true DSQ diapers, buy them from a diaper service or over the Internet.

Shaped, or contoured, diapers have narrow centers and wide wings to fit a baby's shape. They can be pinned, but diaper wraps with Velcro-type closures hold them securely in place. Shaped diapers aren't as versatile as unfolded and prefolded diapers; you'll have to buy at least two sizes before your baby is potty-trained. But these diapers are very easy to use, and when a baby outgrows

Washing Diapers

Your grandmother may have soaked diapers or rinsed them in the toilet, but these measures aren't necessary, at least not today.

You'll need a pail with a lid, such as a foot-operated kitchen garbage pail. If the pail doesn't have a removable liner, you might line the pail with a nylon tote bag (cotton would absorb odors) for carrying the diapers to the washing machine. Wet diapers can go directly into the pail. If diapers are soiled, shake the solids into the toilet, using a bit of toilet paper, if necessary. Whatever is left will come off easily in the wash.

If odors come from the pail, you might sprinkle in ¼ cup of baking soda when the pail is empty, and add a sprinkle on top when the smell gets strong. Or put a couple of drops of tea-tree or lavender oil on a cloth, and drop the cloth into the empty pail (these essential oils are available at most natural-foods stores).

Detergent for diapers should be free of phosphates, to protect waterways, and most parents prefer diapers that are free of fragrances, dyes, and fabric softeners as well. Fabric softeners create a waxy buildup on cloth diapers that cause them to repel urine instead of absorbing it. Don't use "baby soaps" that are advertised as safe for a baby's delicate skin but are full of irritating fragrances.

When it's time to wash the diapers, make sure folded diapers are completely open. Secure Velcro-type tabs (so the hook side doesn't fill with threads and lint), and pull the inserts out of pocket diapers. Run a cold-water cycle using ½ cup of baking soda rather than detergent; this will help keep the diapers white and fresh-smelling. When the cycle has finished, run a hot wash–cold rinse cycle using about half the amount of detergent suggested on the label.

If your water is hard or if you're planning to line-dry the diapers, you might try using vinegar as a water softener. Fill a Downy fabric softener ball (which you can buy in a supermarket) half full of distilled white vinegar, or put the vinegar in the water-softener drawer of your washer. The vinegar should remove all traces of soap and urine and act as a fabric softener. You shouldn't use vinegar, however, with diaper covers, all-in-ones, or pocket diapers made of polyester.

If your washer has a "sanitary" or "super-hot" setting, you can use it instead of a cold cycle followed by a hot one. The sanitary setting provides a very long cycle, lasting one and a half to two hours. If you wash and dry diapers three times before using them, the fibers will swell and fluff and become much more absorbent. If the diapers get dingy over time, use a little color-safe bleach, or hang them in the sun for a safe, natural bleaching.

them they work well as diaper-doublers. You can also use them as inserts in a pocket diaper.

Fitted diapers are made from absorbent fabrics, usually cotton or hemp. These diapers are hourglass-shaped to eliminate folding and are gusseted for a snug fit around the legs. Typically, a soaker pad is either sewn into the diaper or is laid or snapped in with each change. Fitted diapers have attached fasteners, either snaps or Velcro-type closures. Because of the elastic around the legs and waist, fitted diapers prevent leakage better than other cloth diapers do, although they still need an added cover. Like shaped diapers, fitted diapers must be replaced with larger sizes as a baby grows.

An all-in-one combines a fitted diaper with an attached waterproof cover, making a washable diaper that is most like a disposable. All-in-ones are the easiest diapers to use, but also the most expensive. In addition, the waterproof backing makes them harder to clean and more difficult to dry, and blocks air circulation to the baby's skin.

A pocket diaper is like an all-in-one except for the inside pocket, usually made of Micro fleece, in which you place an absorbent hemp insert or a folded or shaped cotton diaper. Provided you remove the insert before doing the laundry, a pocket diaper allows for more thorough cleaning and faster drying than do all-in-one diapers. Both all-in-one and pocket diapers must be replaced with larger sizes as a baby grows.

DIAPER COVERS. Unless you are using an all-in-one or a pocket diaper, you will need some kind of shell over a cloth diaper, to keep *you* dry. Fabrics range from waterproof (polyurethane) to water-resistant (nylon or fleece) to very absorbent (wool).

There are two basic styles of diaper covers: wraps and pull-on pants. A diaper wrap wraps around the diaper, from front to back, and closes with Velcro-type closures or snaps. The snug fit makes it unnecessary to pin or clip the diaper beneath.

Pull-on pants have elastic at the waist and legs. If you use pull-on pants with folded or shaped diapers, you must pin or clip the diaper closed. Generally, the most economical diaper covers are waterproof pull-on pants. These used to be made of plastic that would crack and discolor, but today better synthetic fabrics are used.

BABY-CARE BASICS

There are a lot of little items that you will want to consider getting for the day-to-day care of your baby.

Pacifiers

These are controversial. If pacifiers are used frequently in the early weeks, a baby may have trouble learning to breastfeed. Also, studies have linked pacifier use with ear infections. But babies need a lot of sucking time, and those who aren't given pacifiers or the breast whenever they fuss may come to depend on their fingers or thumbs. Some think that finger- or thumb-sucking is a harder habit to break than sucking on a pacifier.

If you decide to try a pacifier, find one that is made of silicone and orthodontically shaped—that is, shaped to conform to the interior of the mouth.

Bath Items

BABY BATHTUB. Some parents make do by bathing the baby in the kitchen sink or bathing along with the baby in a regular bathtub, but others buy a special little tub for the early months. If you decide to buy one, look for a skid-resistant surface, and also for a drain in the bottom so you won't strain and splash yourself when you empty the tub.

BABY BATH PAD. If you decide to wash the baby in the sink, you might want one of these to keep the baby from slipping. Avoid the kind that are huge sponges; they are difficult to dry, and they breed mold and bacteria.

BATH SEATS AND RINGS. Used when a baby can sit up but can't be trusted to stay up, these give parents a false sense of security. Babies have drowned because their parents have left them unattended in these devices.

BABY SOAP. This tends to be milder than other soaps, with less fragrance and without antibacterial chemicals or abrasives. Mild soaps not especially intended for babies, such as Neutrogena and Dove, are usually kind to a young baby's skin.

BABY SHAMPOO. Generally milder than other shampoos, baby shampoo doesn't sting if it gets in the eyes.

Diapering Items

BABY WIPES. Commercially made disposable wipes are popular, but the perfumes and other chemicals can irritate a baby's skin. Chemical-free baby wipes are available but more expensive. Some parents use soft, dry disposable wipes such as Quickables; these are used in many hospitals and are available through medical suppliers. Other parents use Viva paper towels, which are both soft and strong. You cut the roll in half or quarters with a serrated knife, pull out the tube, and then dampen the towels with water or baby oil.

You can, of course, do without disposable wipes and use cloth instead. Baby washcloths work well; so does cotton flannel or terry, cut into squares. Just moisten the cloths before using them. If you're using cloth diapers, wash the wipes along with the diapers.

DIAPER-RASH OINTMENT. Because urine and acid stools irritate the skin, many babies get diaper rash. A petroleum ointment such as A&D can be used every day to protect your baby's skin. To protect a baby who is especially prone to rash, or to treat an existing rash, use an ointment that contains zinc oxide, a longer-lasting barrier than petroleum. A&D, Balmex, and Desitin all make zinc-oxide ointments.

Medical Items

Included here are first-aid supplies, many of which you may have in your home already. *Note:* Syrup of ipecac and liquefied charcoal are no longer recommended for home use. In the event of poisoning, call a poison-control center.

COTTON SWABS AND ALCOHOL. These are to care for the umbilical cord stump. Swab the cord with alcohol at most diaper changes.

THERMOMETER. The best type is digital. Glass thermometers are no longer recommended because of the danger of leaking mercury; besides, digital thermometers work faster and are much easier to read. Digital thermometers are used with disposable plastic sheaths. A young baby's temperature is taken rectally; you lay the baby face down across your lap and insert the lubricated thermometer ½ inch into the rectum. When a baby reaches three months of age, you can take his temperature by putting the thermometer in his armpit and holding his arm against his side.

PETROLEUM JELLY. This is used as a lubricant for taking a rectal temperature.

NASAL ASPIRATOR AND SALINE DROPS. When your baby has a stuffy nose, you can loosen the mucus by dropping saline solution into the nose. Then you can gently remove the mucus with a small nasal aspirator, a rubber bulb with a narrow tip.

INFANT-STRENGTH ACETAMINOPHEN, LIQUID OR SUPPOSITORIES. This is a pain reliever and fever reducer.

CALIBRATED DROPPER AND MEASURING-POURING SPOON. You'll need these for liquid medicines.

HUMIDIFIER OR VAPORIZER. These help to make breathing easier for baby during respiratory illnesses. Cool-mist humidifiers are now considered safe only if they are ultrasonic, have a particle filter, or are used with distilled water. Vaporizers, which produce a hot vapor, are generally preferred over humidifiers.

ICE PACKS. These are handy for a bang on the head.

HYDROGEN PEROXIDE. A mild antiseptic, hydrogen peroxide is useful for cleaning cuts and scrapes.

ADHESIVE BANDAGES. You'll use these for any number of mishaps.

GAUZE PADS AND FIRST-AID TAPE. These items are necessary for covering larger areas of skin.

ANTIBIOTIC OINTMENT. An important item to have on hand, antibiotic ointment can be applied to cuts and scrapes to help prevent infection.

TWEEZERS. You'll need these to remove splinters or stingers.

FIRST-AID BOOK. A first-aid book is an important resource to keep handy.

EMERGENCY CONTACT LIST. Make sure to include a poison-control number.

Grooming Items

FINE-TOOTHED COMB AND SOFT BRUSH. Although you could use a regular comb and brush, a fine-toothed comb is better for fine baby hair, and a soft brush won't irritate baby's sensitive scalp.

MANICURE ITEMS. You can use baby nail clippers or scissors to trim fingernails and toenails, or you can file the baby's nails with am emery board.

BABY OIL. This is good for massage and also for treating cradle cap, a crusty layer that forms on many babies' scalps because the skin grows faster than it falls off. Massage a few drops of oil into the scalp, and then use a fine-toothed comb or a dry terry washcloth to gently rub the flakes away.

CHAPTER 7

Daytime Gear

There will be times when you need to put your baby down while you tend to other things. You can lay the baby in a bassinet or crib, but she may soon object to the lack of stimulation. So most parents get one or two other pieces of equipment in which to set the baby. The most popular items for this purpose are stationary and bouncing infant seats, infant swings, walkers and stationary entertainers, and playpens (which manufacturers now call "play yards" or "playards").

INFANT SEATS
AND BOUNCERS

Many parents use infant car seats as all-purpose baby seats and carriers. Other kinds of infant seats are more stimulating—they rock or bounce, or they have attached toys to play with. For carrying a baby from place to place, infant car seats are very awkward. Can you imagine carrying around a 20-pound bucket of sand in one hand or on your forearm? This is what it's like to carry a baby in a car seat. It's much more sensible to put the baby into a sling or other soft carrier when you get out of your vehicle. Leave the car seat in the car, and leave your hands free for other things.

You can, of course, carry the empty car seat into the house and later put the baby back into it. But you shouldn't leave a baby in a car seat for many hours each day. Confinement in a car seat limits a baby's movements and thus can delay her muscular and sensory development. The semi-upright sitting position, with hips bent, fails to stimulate the baby's lower brain and so can delay the development of physical coordination. For normal development, a baby needs to spend most of her time in a horizontal position, in someone's arms or lying on a level surface. Besides delaying development, the sitting position puts constant pressure on the back of the baby's head, which is why many babies today have misshapen skulls.

Stationary infant seats meant for home use are often called activity seats, because they come with attached toys. Like a car seat or stroller, an activity seat puts the baby in a sitting position. You'll want to take care to limit the total time your baby spends sitting up in any of these seats.

A bouncer seat is a much better place to leave a baby for extended periods. A baby-size sling chair on a slightly inclined frame, the seat bounces when the baby moves. Some bouncer seats can be adjusted to sit the baby upright, but the flat position is best. Many bouncer seats now come with toy bars, vibrators, carrying handles, music boxes, and canopies. Since the seat is usable for only a few months, you may want to consider carefully before paying for more than the basic bouncer. (An extra feature many parents like is the vibrator, which makes the baby feel as if she were riding in a car. Not all babies like this feature, though.) A bouncer seat is a good item to borrow as long as the straps and buckles are in good order.

If you put your baby in an infant seat of any type, never set the seat on a table or countertop. Even if strapped in, older babies sometimes tip themselves over while sitting in stationary infant seats. And because bouncer seats are very lightweight, they are prone to falling off surfaces. Infant seats belong on the floor.

Whether or not you get an infant seat of one sort or another, you'll occasionally want to put your baby on a blanket on the floor. Now that young babies are always put to sleep on their backs (to lessen the risk of Sudden Infant Death Syndrome), short wakeful periods on the stomach help in the development of head and neck control and motor skills.

SWINGS

· ·

Most, though not all, babies enjoy the perpetual motion of a swing. Infant swings come in two types, cranked and battery-operated. The cranked types run for 10 to 30 minutes before they must be cranked again. Parents much prefer the more expensive battery-operated swings, which run until they are shut off and generally make less noise. Like other baby gear, swings come with options: music, toys, variable speeds, sound effects that the baby can activate, storage baskets, side-to-side motion, cradle attachments, and remote control. If a swing doesn't have a cradle attachment, a reclining feature is important, because young babies shouldn't spend much time in the upright position.

Since a bouncer seat and a swing are very similar in function, you probably won't want to buy both. Swings seem to be more effective in buying parents free time, which is why some people

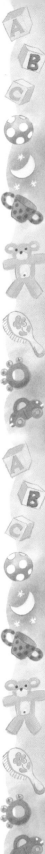

call them "neglect-o-matics." Perhaps because they are such stimulating baby sitters, swings are among the types of baby gear most associated with infant injuries. Parents should use the safety belt, stay in the room when the baby swings, and stop using the swing when the baby reaches 25 pounds.

If you'd like to have an infant swing, you may want to find out whether you can borrow one, since a baby swing is useful for only about six months. After that, a baby is more interested in crawling than swinging.

WALKERS AND STATIONARY ENTERTAINERS

A walker is a baby seat on wheels. Operated by a baby's feet, a walker gives upright mobility to a baby who can't walk on her own. Though still sold in stores, walkers are going out of vogue because they are associated with infant injuries. The most common of these accidents occur when a baby in a walker falls down stairs. Besides being dangerous, a walker can delay a baby's development, especially in learning to walk independently.

Stationary entertainers or "activity centers" have gained popularity as walkers have lost it. A swivel seat suspended over a stationary base, an entertainer has either a flat base with springs that bounce or a curved base that rocks. A baby can sit or stand in the entertainer and play with the attached toys, some of which emit sounds and light, although most babies quickly get bored with these things. Like walkers, entertainers take up quite a bit of room and get bad reviews from child-development experts, who say that these entertainment centers cause developmental delays when used for long periods. If I haven't convinced you not to get an entertainer, consider borrowing rather than buying one, and make it a family policy not to park the baby in it for longer than 20 minutes.

PLAY YARDS
(PLAYPENS)

. . . .

An enclosed space for a baby or toddler to play or sleep in, a play yard is the modern, metal-and-mesh version of the old-fashioned wood-framed playpen. A play yard folds up compactly for storage or travel. With the optional bassinet and changing table that attach to the top rails, a play yard can double as a satellite nursery in a baby's first three or four months. Other options include wheels, toy pockets, a rocking or vibrating mechanism for the bassinet, a sunshade, and mosquito netting.

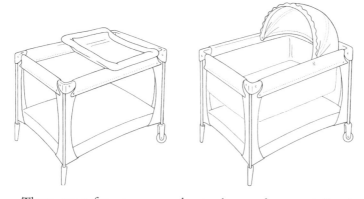

There are safety concerns about play yards, especially those manufactured before 2000. If you consider buying or borrowing a used play yard, make sure it has a mechanism that prevents accidental collapse. With any play yard, remove the changing table before putting the baby inside; otherwise, the baby's head could become entrapped between the table and the rail. Make sure the mattress is securely attached to the floor of the play yard, so the baby can't get trapped between the two. With a used play yard, it's a good idea to replace the mattress. Stop using your play yard when a baby reaches 30 pounds or attempts to climb out.

CHAPTER 8

Traveling with Your Baby

A great variety of infant gear is intended to make it easier to carry a baby, on foot or in a car. In this chapter I'll tell you how to choose and install a car seat, how to make sense of all the options for wearing your baby (in a front pack, backpack, or sling), and how to decide whether you need a stroller and which sort suits you best.

CAR SEATS

. . . .

By law, infants and small children must be strapped into a safety-approved car seat when riding in a vehicle. Car seats manufactured today are all safety-approved by the U.S. government.

A car seat sold secondhand may not meet current safety standards. Hidden damage from a crash could make the seat unsafe. Or the model could have been recalled; nearly every brand of car seat has been subject to recalls in the past. Often, the manufacturer's instructions are missing from used car seats.

Borrowing or accepting a hand-me-down car seat from a friend or family member can be risky as well. If the seat is older than six years, it probably doesn't meet current standards. If you decide to use a secondhand car seat, make sure that is it not more than two years old, that the model is still in production and has not been recalled, and that you have the installation instructions. You might call the manufacturer to order a new set of installation instructions and ask about any recall. You can also find out about recalls by calling the National Highway Traffic Safety Administration at 888-327-4236.

If you cannot afford a new car seat, you might also check around for a free car-seat loaner program. Most hospitals and health departments know about these programs.

Before you buy a car seat, make sure it is compatible with your car. To check on the compatibility between various car seats and vehicles, consult the Web site www.carseatdata.org. If you buy a new car seat, send in the warranty and registration form so that you will be likely to get any recall notice. Before you buy, also consider which type of car seat you want. For infants, there are two types to choose from: infant seats and convertible infant-toddler seats.

Infant Car Seats

These rear-facing, semi-reclined bucket seats are used for infants up to about 20 pounds or about 26 inches in height. Infant seats fit young babies better than convertible infant-toddler seats and are proven to be safer, because they cradle babies more securely.

Most infant seats today snap in and out of a base that is installed in the vehicle. This allows you to get a sleeping baby out of the car without waking him. If you want to use one seat in two or more vehicles, you can buy extra bases. Some of these seats snap into a stroller. Many parents use the snap-in seats as general-purpose infant seats and as hand carriers, although their weight and bulkiness make carrying them difficult. But a baby should not spend any more time in a car seat than is necessary, because confinement in the semi-sitting position can adversely affect infant development.

Some infant seats buckle directly onto the seat of a car. These are easier to use if you travel by cab or in other people's cars. Every infant car seat has a harness, a set of straps that hold the baby in. The harness can be one of two types, three-point or five-point. The three-point harness has two adjustable shoulder belts that snap into a lock between the baby's legs. The five-point harness adds two other straps, which fit over the baby's thighs to restrain the hips. The three-point harness is much easier to use, but the five-point harness fits babies better and offers more protection. A five-point harness is essential for a young baby born prematurely.

When shopping for an infant car seat, look for a harness that is easy to adjust. Some car-seat models require an adjustment from behind the seat to tighten or loosen the harness over the baby's shoulders. Adjusting the harness is much easier when the mechanism for this is at the front of the seat.

The harness should always extend from the seat back at or just below the level of the baby's shoulders. As the baby grows, the harness level should be raised. To allow this, a car seat should have multiple harness slots. Also, changing the height of the harness will be much easier if there is an automatic height adjuster in the front of the seat. Otherwise you'll have to rethread the harness through the back. The harness may come together over the baby's chest with a sliding clip or a snap. A snap is the safer option. The best infant car seats come with firm, thick harness straps that are difficult to twist. This avoids the problem of worn, flimsy straps that become difficult to use.

When an infant seat is installed in a car, its base should be level. Leveling is easiest if the seat has a lever for raising and lowering the base. Also helpful is a level indicator on the side of the base.

An infant car seat should be retired when your baby meets either the weight or height limit recommended by the manufacturer. At this point, you'll need to get a convertible infant-toddler seat.

Convertible Infant-Toddler Seats

Convertible seats are used for infants and toddlers up to 40 pounds. Until a baby reaches a certain weight and height, a convertible seat is used in a semi-reclining, rear-facing position. Then the seat is turned upright and face forward until the child has outgrown it. Generally, the baby must be one year old and at least 20 pounds in weight before the seat is turned front-facing. Keeping a baby rear-facing until this point helps prevent whiplash in the event that the car stops suddenly. Some manufacturers make seats that can be used rear-facing until a child reaches 30 or 35 pounds.

If you're attracted by the idea of buying just one car seat that can be used from birth through preschool, you may want to think again. Convertible seats aren't as safe for young babies as infant seats are, and many parents find convertible seats less convenient in the early months.

Whether you get a convertible seat now or wait until your baby is a toddler, you should know that these seats come with any of three types of harness systems: three-point, five-point, and bar shield. A five-point restraint provides the most protection in the event of a crash. Seats with a bar shield, a solid bar that comes down over the child's head, are no longer recommended.

The height of the harness should be easily adjustable if you'll use the car seat in the rear-facing position. When the seat is turned front-facing, only the top harness slot should be used, since generally it is the only one sufficiently reinforced to withstand the force of a crash in the face-forward position.

Another good car-seat feature is a machine-washable seat cover that is easy to remove and replace. New seat covers can be ordered from some car-seat makers, and several online companies sell washable covers that fit most brands of seats.

Other helpful features are a reclining foot on the front of the seat, a front-adjustable harness, and firm, thick harness straps that snap together over the chest.

Installing Your Car Seat

After you buy a car seat, you'll want to install it right away to make sure that it will work with your vehicle. Read both the instructions that came with the car seat and the relevant instructions in your vehicle's owner's manual. If you are missing either set of instructions, call the manufacturer for a new set.

Ideally, the car seat should go in the center of the vehicle's back seat, the safest place in the car. If this is not possible, use one of the rear window seats. A car seat should never be installed in front of an air bag. If the car seat must go in a seat with an air bag, have the air bag deactivated.

All car seats manufactured since 2002 come with the LATCH or the ISOFIX system. This means that the car seat has straps or rigid connectors that connect to anchor bars in the lower seat back of the car rather than to the car's seat belt. Most newer vehicles have the corresponding LATCH or ISOFIX anchor bars; check your vehicle's owner's manual to see whether it does. These systems make car-seat installation both easier and safer. If your car has no anchor bars, you can install the car seat using the vehicle's safety belts.

Older cars without the LATCH system may have safety belts that lock only on sudden impact. These will not keep a car seat secure unless a locking clip is attached to keep the belt tight all the time. Car seats come with these locking clips. A vehicle made after 1995 may have a safety-lock feature that makes a locking clip unnecessary. The new LATCH system eliminates the need for any locking clip, because the system doesn't use vehicle safety belts.

A car seat must be installed so that it inclines at the angle recommended by the manufacturer. An infant seat will incline at the right angle if the base is leveled. A leveling lever and level indicator usually make this easy. In some cars, though, installing a rear-facing car seat is difficult because the seat of the vehicle slopes too much. You may have to level the surface by placing padding underneath the car seat.

Convertible infant-toddler car seats come with a tether at the top of the seat that attaches to the rear of the vehicle. When the seat is used front-facing, the tether prevents the seat from pitching forward in a sudden stop. Most new vehicles come with an anchor bolt to which you can snap the tether. An older vehicle may need to have an anchor bolt installed. Some auto dealers will do this without charge.

When you've installed the car seat, shake it hard. It should not move more than an inch in either direction. To make sure you've installed the seat correctly, have it checked by a child passenger safety (CPS) technician. These inspections are free. You can probably find a CPS technician in your community by contacting your local health department or highway police department. Chrysler dealerships offer free car-seat inspections, too, regardless of the model of the vehicle. And the National Highway Traffic Safety Administration maintains a list of CPS locations on its Web site, www.nhtsa.dot.gov.

Accessories for Car Travel

Here are some items that you may consider buying along with a car seat. An infant headrest is a U-shaped pillow that fits into the car seat to keep the baby's head from rolling from side to side (a rolled-up towel or receiving blanket can accomplish the same thing). Also available are neck supports that hold a baby's head upright while he naps. Roll-down shades for the car windows are helpful in keeping the sun off the baby. Seat protectors are mats that are placed under the car seat to prevent soiling of the vehicle seat. Because dressing a baby in bulky clothing does not allow her to be snugly strapped into her car seat, you can buy an infant-seat cover that fits around both the baby and the seat to provide warmth (a heavy blanket works as well).

Some car-seat accessories should be avoided. A mirror that attaches to the back seat of a car lets you observe a rear-facing baby in the back seat through the rear-view mirror, but these mirrors could become dangerous in the event of a crash. Likewise, toy bars that are positioned in front of a baby could be hazardous during a sudden stop. Strap covers that pad the car-seat harness may also pose a danger, if they keep the harness from fitting the baby snugly. Lastly, still available are seat-belt tighteners that were used to tighten vehicle belts before the introduction of the LATCH system. These tighteners are now thought by safety experts to be dangerous, because they mislead parents into thinking that any poor-fitting car seat can be made to fit properly with one of these devices.

SOFT STRAP-ON CARRIERS AND SLINGS

. . . .

Wearing your baby is a wonderful way to keep her happy and close to you while keeping your arms free. A wearable carrier spares you the hassle of strollers and allows you to go places where strollers can't. Wearing your baby can give you peace, too, because babies carried against their parents' bodies cry less. Indoors as well as out, you can comfort your baby against your body while tending to other things. Learning how to put the carrier on, take it off, and get the baby into it may require a little practice.

Front Strap-on Carriers

These are pouches that hold an infant in an upright position against the wearer's chest. Front strap-on carriers are probably the most popular wearable carriers among U.S. parents. In the early weeks, the baby faces the wearer's chest with his legs suspended through leg openings. Later, as the baby gets more head and neck control, he can usually be turned to face outward. Because the straps are adjustable, either parent can use the same carrier. Strap-on carriers are a little complicated to put on, because the straps must be crossed in the back and secured in the front. This is difficult to do while carrying a baby in one arm.

Although manufacturers suggest that front carriers can be worn until a baby reaches 25 to 40 pounds, parents often complain of shoulder and back discomfort at far less weight. A padded belt can minimize discomfort by distributing the weight to the hips. Here are other features to look for in a front strap-on carrier:

- ◆ Soft, washable fabric
- ◆ Wide, thick, padded shoulder straps
- ◆ A sturdy support for the baby's head
- ◆ An adjustable seat, so you can wear your baby at a comfortable level as he grows
- ◆ Pockets for carrying things
- ◆ Buckles that are easy to use but require two motions to undo
- ◆ Snaps that unfasten only with a strong pull

If you inherit a used front carrier, examine it to make sure that all the belts and buckles are in good working order and that there are no tears around the snaps. If the carrier is a Baby Björn made between 1991 and 1998, be aware that the model was recalled because the leg openings were too large; small babies could fall through. For a free retrofit kit that rectifies the problem, call the company at 877-242-5676.

Front-back Strap-on Carriers

Some soft carriers can be used on the back as well as the front. Many parents find that carriers worn on the back are much more comfortable and also safer, since they keep babies away from hot stoves and other dangers. One brand of front-back carrier is the Ergo (see Other Resources for New Parents, page 147). Chinese-style baby carriers are also becoming popular in the United States. A Chinese-style carrier consists of a rectangular seat area with four straps, two that tie around the wearer's waist and two that go over the shoulders. Used for centuries by Chinese women, these carriers, worn on the front or back, are great for babies of all ages.

Slings

Used since ancient times, baby slings are still worn around the world. They have become increasingly popular in the United States since William Sears, a pediatrician and an author, began recommending them for the practice of "attachment parenting," his term for keeping a baby close and content. Parents who practice attachment parenting feel strongly that it enhances the bond between parent and baby.

A sling is basically a length of fabric wrapped over the wearer's shoulder and draped across the chest to create a hammock for the baby. Your baby can lie in a sling as he would if cradled in your arms. When he is older, he can sit facing outward, straddle your hip, or ride on your back. Fans of slings feel that they let babies be carried in more natural positions than allowed by a front pack, which forces a baby's legs apart. Women say that slings are great for supporting a baby during breastfeeding and for protecting a nursing mother's privacy.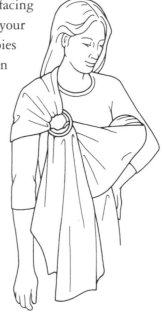

Slings require more practice in putting on and settling the baby into than front packs do. When you buy a sling, ask to be shown how to wear it, or get a lesson from a friend who is a sling user. If you can't get a hands-on lesson, consult the written instructions that come with all slings. Some sling makers even offer a video to show parents how to wear their baby.

The simplest sling is a length of fabric wrapped around the baby and tied. Other slings are made to size; you choose one according to your T-shirt size. In this case, a couple may find that they need two slings. Some slings have padded shoulders, but the unpadded ones tend to be just as comfortable and less bulky. Most slings with shoulder padding also have a double set of rings for adjusting the size. The best fit places the baby close to the wearer's waist.

FRAME BACKPACKS

These are useful from the time a baby can sit unsupported, usually after six months of age, until she grows into a child who can manage long walks on her own. Baby backpacks can go where strollers can't, such as on hiking trails, and many families prefer them to strollers even for city walks.

Whedn wearing a baby either in a soft strap-on carrier or a sling, there are a few rules to keep in mind: Never wear a baby while drinking hot beverages or cooking at the stove unless the baby is on your back. When you reach down for something, bend at the knees instead of at the waist. Do not wear a baby when biking or skating. Lastly, never wear the baby in a car instead of using a car seat.

A frame backpack consists of a fabric seat for the baby suspended inside a plastic, aluminum, or steel frame. A kick stand allows the pack to sit firmly on the ground while the baby is installed in the seat or removed. A padded hip belt, provided on better-made packs, distributes the weight from the wearer's shoulders to the hips.

To put on the backpack, stand it on the ground and put the baby into the seat. Then squat down, lift the backpack onto your shoulders, fasten the hip belt, and pull the stand against your back.

Backpacks come in a wide range of prices. The best and most expensive ones are made by manufacturers of hiking equipment. If you and your partner are serious hikers, you will most likely want a high-end model. Low-end carriers are fine for short outings.

When shopping for a backpack, look for thick and adjustable shoulder straps and an adjustable, padded hip belt. Pick a durable fabric that is easy to sponge-clean. Make sure the straps and buckles are easy to adjust but require two motions to do so. Any snaps should take strong force to undo. An adjustable seat lets the baby be carried lower as he grows taller. A harness or belt should be provided to keep the baby from climbing out, or from falling out if the parent trips or falls. Try out the pack you're considering with the baby in it, if possible, to make sure that it is comfortable for both of you.

It's fine to use a secondhand backpack as long as it is in good shape, with no rips in the fabric and with straps and belts in good working order.

STROLLERS AND CARRIAGES

. . . .

A stroller or carriage may be a must-have for you, especially if you live in the heart of a city or have a bad back. Even if you live beyond the sidewalks and don't mind carrying a baby, a stroller can be used as a portable seat indoors as well as outdoors. A carriage, or a stroller that converts into a carriage, can also be used as a portable bed.

But strollers can be a hassle if pavement is lacking and wheelchair ramps are nonexistent. In any crowded area, a stroller is a nuisance. Pushing one out into traffic is dangerous, especially if you're entering the crosswalk from behind a parked car. If you are content to carry your baby in a sling, front pack, or backpack, you may not need a stroller at all, or at least you may be able to get by with an inexpensive one.

You may be surprised to learn that there are eight different types of strollers. Before you choose a particular model, decide which type best meets your needs. You may have difficulty settling on a type, because the perfect stroller has yet to be designed.

Carriages

Also called prams, these are bassinets on large wheels for strolling in style with young babies. Usually the infant lies flat on a comfortable mattress, although in some carriages the mattress can be raised for sitting up. A carriage has plenty of space for bundling a baby in cold weather and a generous hood for protecting a baby from the sun. Sometimes the basket can be removed to serve as a bassinet. If not, the carriage itself can serve as a rolling bassinet in the home.

Carriages have some disadvantages. They are quite expensive. They are heavy, usually about 30 pounds, and they do not fold up. Because the front wheels are fixed, carriages are difficult to turn, especially in tight areas.

If you'd like to use a secondhand pram, consider ordering a new mattress.

Convertible Carriage-Strollers

One of these fulfills two functions: It is a carriage for an infant to lie in and a stroller for an older baby or toddler to sit up in. A reversible handlebar allows the carriage to be pushed with the baby facing the parent, and then switched so that the baby faces outward in the stroller. Many of these strollers have a full hood for protection from the elements.

Parents who do a great deal of walking may prefer these heavy, well-made strollers over conventional kinds, but convertible strollers can be difficult to fold and carry. They can also be hard to find, because many manufacturers have replaced them with "travel systems" (see page 102). Borrowing a carriage-stroller in good working order is a great option.

Conventional Strollers

In this category are strollers ranging from no-frills to very luxurious. Some are lightweight, less than 15 pounds. Some are heavy-duty. A few can be used with newborns; some of the more expensive ones allow an infant car seat to be snapped onto the top. But most of these strollers are upright, made for older babies who can sit unsupported. Most conventional strollers are easy to fold and to set up.

UMBRELLA STROLLERS. These lightweight strollers are named for the shape they take when folded. Most are very inexpensive and cheaply made. Their small wheels make an umbrella stroller difficult to push over anything but smooth pavement or flooring, although some more expensive models have pivoting front wheels for better maneuvering. Few models have features like full sun hoods or baskets, and hanging a bag on a handlebar can cause umbrella strollers to tip backward. Because the cloth sling seats lack head support, these strollers are inappropriate for young babies. Still, umbrella strollers are handy for traveling if you get tired of carrying your baby.

TRAVEL SYSTEMS. These combine a car seat and a stroller. The infant carrier serves as a rear-facing car seat until you're ready for a

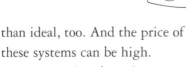

walk, and then it attaches to the stroller to serve as a carriage. When the baby outgrows the infant seat, you can place her directly into the stroller. On the downside, most of these strollers are bulky and heavy; they may weigh as much as 30 pounds. Some parents end up abandoning the stroller for lighter equipment. Many complain that the car seat is less

than ideal, too. And the price of these systems can be high.

A similar but less expensive option is a stroller base, a frame on wheels to which you snap a car seat to make a small reclined stroller, usually with a roomy storage basket beneath. Most but not

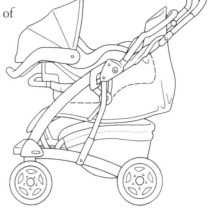

all infant car seats fit into a particular stroller-base model. At a cost of about $50, a stroller base can be used until the baby outgrows the car seat, between six months and one year. Some higher-end conventional strollers also allow an infant car seat to be snapped on.

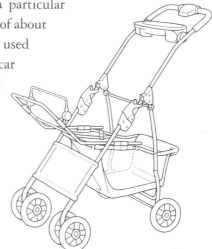

Stroller base

JOGGING STROLLERS. These three-wheeled strollers are designed to carry babies and young children while their parents run, jog, or walk. A sling seat holds the baby. Fixed bicycle-style wheels—large for running, and medium or small for jogging or walking—are attached to a plastic, steel, or aluminum frame. Steel joggers are the heaviest and can rust; aluminum frames are recommended if the stroller is to be used for running or jogging. Generally, there are two kinds of brakes: handlebar brakes to slow and stop the stroller, and a foot-operated brake for parking. Because these strollers can speed along at close to 15 miles per hour, a tether strap is provided to keep parent and stroller connected in case the parent loses his grip.

The big advantage of a jogging stroller is the smooth ride it provides over unpaved areas such as gravel, sand, or grass. Still, the jostling of the ride may be too much for a baby less than six months old or unable to sit unsupported. And there are disadvantages to these strollers: They require a lot of space; they can tip when the back wheels are raised over a curb or other obstacle; the tubes can puncture and develop slow leaks; the tires may have to be removed for storage; and the fixed wheels make the strollers difficult to steer and maneuver on city sidewalks and indoors.

ALL-TERRAIN OR SPORT-UTILITY STROLLERS. These are the most recent type of stroller on the market. Advertised for use

Stroller Buying

Here are some things to consider when shopping for a stroller:

♦ Often the handles are too low. Some strollers have handles that can be adjusted for height, but very tall parents may find that the highest setting is not high enough. Parents with a long stride may find that they continually bump into the underside of a stroller. Walking with the stroller across a store may help you weed out ones that simply don't fit.

♦ Some strollers have two handles; others have a single handlebar. Single-bar strollers are generally easier to steer with one hand. Two-handled strollers require both hands to maneuver, but they also fold more compactly.

♦ Stroller wheels are often a problem. Cheap plastic wheels generally work poorly. A stroller will ride more smoothly and maneuver better if it has double wheels on each leg and if at least the front wheels swivel. Generally, larger wheels offer a smoother ride but take up more space when the stroller is folded.

♦ The best strollers are easy to fold and set up. One-handed mechanisms are best. Try folding and setting up the stroller before you buy it.

♦ When the stroller is folded, consider its size. Will it fit in the trunk of the car?

♦ The weight of the stroller may also factor into your choice. A lightweight stroller is best if you will be lifting and carrying it a lot. Umbrella strollers are usually the lightest in weight, but most aren't very durable. Aluminum strollers are lighter than steel ones but generally more expensive. Aluminum may be worth the extra cost, however, because steel strollers are prone to rusting. Extra features add to a stroller's weight.

◆ A reclining seat is more comfortable when the baby or toddler falls asleep in the stroller. The reclining mechanism should be easy to use.

◆ Well-padded seats instead of simple cardboard ones are not only nicer for lengthy stroller trips but also add comfort to the back of the baby's legs, which will be unsupported until they grow long enough to reach the footrests.

◆ Seat cushions or covers should be removable for machine washing.

◆ A small overhead shade may not be enough to keep the sun off of your baby. You may prefer a full sun canopy, or you can buy a separate sunshade.

◆ An under-stroller basket will be handy if you will be taking the stroller shopping or on errands. Make sure the basket is fully accessible when the stroller seat is reclined or when the car seat is attached.

◆ Some strollers come with rain covers, but if yours doesn't you can buy one separately.

◆ Some strollers come with a handlebar tray and cup holder for the parent. These add extra weight. You can buy a clip-on cup holder if you need one.

◆ Some strollers come with front trays for the baby.

STROLLER BUYING, continued

- ◆ The front bar should be padded for the baby's safety. So you can get the baby out easily when she gets big, the bar should also be removable.

- ◆ Safety belts should be provided. A five-point harness is most protective.

- ◆ At least two of the wheels should have brakes.

- ◆ You'll want to check whether the stroller has been approved as safe by the Juvenile Products Manufacturers Association (JPMA). The certification will be on either the stroller or the box it comes in.

---

on rough terrain, including uneven sidewalks, all-terrain strollers have three or four large air-filled wheels. These strollers generally cost less than joggers and offer features joggers don't, such as reclining seats, canopies, and shock absorbers. All-terrains are wider than most other strollers and tend to be more difficult to maneuver, especially if the front wheels are fixed.

MULTI-SEAT STROLLERS. These are used for young siblings, twins, and shared child care. For a full description, see page 120.

Stroller Accessories

There are several items you might consider buying to go along with your stroller. If you think that you may stroll in the rain or snow, you might get either a rain cover or a "boot," a fabric flap that connects to the stroller and covers the baby's lower body. For warmth in cold weather, you can buy a wearable heavy bag that straps to the stroller (a thick blanket can accomplish the same thing, but unless you tuck it in well behind the baby it may fall on the ground).

Sunshades and mosquito netting are available for strollers, too. So are clip-on holders for your drinking cup, and mesh bags that hang on the back of a stroller for storing things. You can also buy handlebar extenders. These add several inches to the handle height, but unfortunately they may make the stroller difficult to fold.

BIKING EQUIPMENT

If you have been looking forward to biking with your baby, you will have to wait a while. Bicycle trailers should be used only after a child starts walking, when he is old enough to withstand the motion. Mounted bicycle seats are also unsafe for younger babies. Appropriately sized biking helmets are unavailable for children less than a year old.

When considering biking equipment to use with your toddler, keep in mind that a trailer is not necessarily safer than a mounted bicycle seat. A trailer is not always visible to drivers, and it can tip over if the bike is abruptly turned. Safety experts recommend that bicycle trailers be used only off streets and on smooth surfaces.

If you'd prefer a mounted bicycle seat over a trailer, get a seat with a five-point harness (with straps over both shoulders and hips), adjustable footrests, and a high backrest. When you ride, keep in mind that a mounted bicycle seat makes the bicycle less stable. In either a trailer or a mounted bicycle seat, a toddler should wear a fitted helmet.

DIAPER BAGS

Your diaper bag not only hauls all of your baby's supplies when you are out of the house, but it also may turn into a second purse, holding things like car keys, a wallet, and sunglasses. Some parents

WHAT TO PUT IN

Your Diaper Bag

- ◆ Several diapers and a changing pad
- ◆ Baby wipes and diaper cream
- ◆ A receiving blanket
- ◆ A change of clothes
- ◆ A plastic bag for wet things
- ◆ A hat for the sun, cold, or both
- ◆ Sunscreen, if the baby is older than six months
- ◆ Bottles of formula, if the baby is bottle-fed
- ◆ Small toys

have two diaper bags, a smaller one for quick trips and a larger one for longer outings.

Diaper bags come in all sizes and shapes, but most come in one of two styles, tote or backpack. Many parents prefer backpacks because they are more comfortable to carry for long distances or when pushing a stroller. Many backpack diaper bags, however, have only one narrow top opening, which means that items at the bottom of the bag may be difficult to reach. An ordinary backpack made for school or day hikes may have more convenient openings and compartments. A good backpack conforms well to the wearer's body and has wide, padded straps that adjust for the best fit.

A tote should have a handle for carrying by hand as well as a strap long enough to go over your head and shoulder. An ordinary satchel may have as many useful features as one made for baby things.

Whichever style of bag you prefer, there are several features you will want to look for:

◆ The fabric should be tear-resistant and easy to clean. Vinyl and quilted cloth bags are less durable than heavy-duty nylon and other woven synthetic fabrics such as microfiber. The bag's interior should be made of a washable fabric as well.

◆ So you'll have no trouble finding things in the bag, look for compartments on the inside and out. Inside compartments should be see-through. Outside pockets are handy for items that you'll reach for often, such as keys.

◆ A waterproof pouch for wet things is a nice accessory, but you can use any sealable plastic bag for the same purpose.

◆ If you will be carrying bottles, you'll appreciate an insulated storage pocket.

◆ A cushioned changing pad can be helpful; if one doesn't come with the bag, you can purchase a pad separately.

CHAPTER 9

Getting Ready to Feed Solid Foods

Breast milk or formula is all your baby will need for about the first six months. After that, you can begin introducing solids.

BEST BOOK ABOUT FEEDING SOLIDS

Child of Mine: Feeding with Love and Good Sense, by Ellyn Satter (see The Parenting Bookshelf, page 143)

LEARN ABOUT FEEDING SOLIDS

In the beginning, offer solid foods right after breastfeeding or formula feeding, because milk will be your baby's most valuable food until she is well established on table foods. Start with soft, puréed foods, such as iron-fortified cereal. When your baby can manage cereal and other puréed food, you can begin offering foods with a little more texture, such as table foods mashed with a fork. You can start helping your baby learn to drink from a cup at about six months of age, too.

HIGHCHAIRS, BOOSTER SEATS, AND CLIP-ON SEATS

Highchairs

You don't need to shop for a highchair until your baby is about six months old and ready to join the family for meals. Even then, your baby may protest at being put into a highchair. You may find it easier to hold the baby on your lap, at least for the first few weeks of feeding solids.

Highchairs come in a variety of styles, with features that may or may not be important for you and your baby. The classic wooden highchair is less popular now than highchairs made of metal or plastic. Wooden chairs lack some modern features such as foldability, height adjustability, padded seating, and rolling casters. Still, wooden chairs have been used for generations, and many parents find them more pleasing to the eye than modern highchairs.

If you are considering using an older wooden highchair, check the finish on the tray. Even if the finish on the rest of the chair is in good condition, the tray may need stripping, sanding, and refinishing. Use a water-based finish.

If you would prefer a plastic or metal-framed chair, there are several features you will want to consider. Most of these chairs provide adjustable height settings. Two heights, one for feeding the baby while using the tray and another for pushing the chair up to the family table, are probably all you need. Some chairs also have a reclining feature, so that a baby too young to sit up can join the family during mealtimes.

Some highchairs can be folded for compact storage. If you plan to use this feature often, make sure that the folding mechanism is easy to manage. When a folded chair is opened, it should automatically lock to prevent collapse. Casters on the legs are important if you think you will want to move the chair often—from the kitchen to the dining room, for example. The addition of casters tends to make highchairs larger. If you want to be able to wheel a chair around, make sure the casters can be locked.

The tray of the highchair is another consideration. You should be able to attach and remove it easily with just one hand. A baby, however, should not be able to do this. Some trays have a side-release mechanism that is easy for a baby to manipulate, causing the tray to fall off. Other chairs have a pull release under the tray, where the baby can kick it loose. Check to make sure that any chair you are considering has either a kick guard or a push-button release to prevent this from happening. Also make sure that the tray isn't too high for a baby's comfort or so far from the seat back that there would be a large gap between the baby and her meal. You can check this with a measuring tape: The tray should be no more than 8 inches from the seat and 7 inches from the seat back when the tray is in its closest position.

The seat of the highchair should be padded and covered with vinyl so that it's easy to wipe clean, or it should have a removable, washable seat cover. Check the seams for caverns in which food can get trapped.

Babies often get injured by falling or slipping out of highchairs. For this reason, the Juvenile Products Manufacturers Association (JPMA) certifies that highchairs meet basic safety requirements. Look for the JPMA certification sticker on the chair or the box that it comes in. A new highchair should have a crotch post, attached to the tray or to the seat, to prevent a baby from slipping down under the tray. It is better to have the post attached to the seat, so the post can function if the chair is pushed up to a table without the tray.

Keep in mind that most injuries related to highchairs involve the misuse or nonuse of the seat's restraining system. The best restraints are three-point or five-point (over the shoulders or over both shoulders and hips); these prevent the baby from standing up or climbing out of the chair. Most important, never leave your baby unattended in a highchair.

Borrowing or accepting a hand-me-down highchair may be a good idea if the chair seems safe and in good condition. Make sure that the restraints and the tray are in working order.

Booster Seats

A booster seat sits on a regular chair to lift an older baby or toddler to table level. Some booster seats come with removable trays for use away from a table, but these seats aren't ideal substitutes for a highchair; their trays tend to be small and unstable. A toddler,

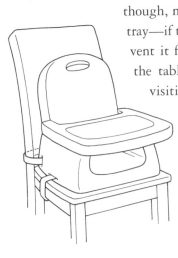

though, may prefer a booster seat—without a tray—if the arms of the family highchair prevent it from being pulled completely up to the table. Booster seats are also useful for visiting and for restaurant meals, because restaurant-owned highchairs and booster seats may not have adequate restraints.

When shopping for a booster seat, look for one that has three straps: one that secures the seat to the chair back, one that secures it to the chair seat, and one that restrains the baby. The bottom of the seat should be rubberized to keep the booster from sliding on the chair.

Clip-on Seats

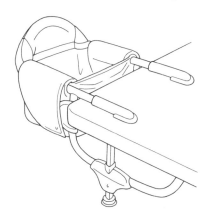

These seats clip onto the edge of a table so the baby can eat with the family. Like boosters, clip-on seats are intended for babies who can sit well unsupported. Unfortunately, these seats can't be attached to some tables, and on others, such as any made of glass, the seats are considered unsafe. Many of these seats fold flat for travel and storage.

FEEDING UTENSILS AND OTHER ACCESSORIES

Many babies receive metal spoons, cups, and bowls as treasured gifts at birth. Traditional baby spoons made of stainless steel, silver, or pewter are fine for feeding your baby. When you first begin offering solid foods, though, you may want to have a few long-handled, small-bowled infant feeding spoons. Many parents prefer those with a protective coating that is soft on the baby's tender gums. Some of these spoons turn color if the food is too hot, but this feature is really unnecessary.

The most practical feeding bowls are made of plastic and have a handle. Some parents opt for a water-heated bowl to keep the food warm longer (you fill the lower section with hot water before putting food into the bowl). When the baby is feeding herself, a bowl with suction cups will help prevent it from ending up on the floor.

The best cup for teaching drinking skills is an ordinary unbreakable, unspouted one. The parent must hold the cup and supervise each and every sip, of course, or the liquid ends up spilled. A cup designed for a baby to hold herself is called a training cup or sippy cup. A sippy cup has a lid with a hard or soft spout that the baby sucks on. Some sippy cups are spill-proof, but the baby must learn how to suck from the spout to get a drink.

Intended to protect the baby's clothing from food stains, bibs are made from a variety of materials, including terry cloth, vinyl, nylon, and hard, molded plastic. Most parents find that bibs with a Velcro or snap closure behind the neck are easier to manage than those with ties.

Especially if the baby will be fed on a carpeted area, you will want to protect the floor with a plastic tablecloth or splash mat. Splash mats are sold at baby supply stores.

Many foods can be easily mashed with a fork, but others may need to be puréed, especially when your baby first begins eating solids. A manual baby-food grinder is an inexpensive, portable tool for this purpose. Certainly, a food processor can do the same thing with just a little more hassle, but processors are inconvenient for preparing the very small amounts of food that a baby needs for one meal. If you have a processor, you might use it for preparing larger quantities of food, which you can then freeze in small portions.

A product for self-feeding is called the Safe Feeder. It consists of a soft mesh bag attached to a handle. Foods that might pose a choking hazard are placed in the bag, and the baby chews on the bag. Some parents put cold fruits in the bag for teething relief. Critics of this gadget feel that chewing on the fabric does not teach self-feeding skills, and that choking can be avoided by offering only soft and non-crumbly food until the baby learns to chew and swallow, and by supervising the baby during meals and snacks.

CHAPTER 10

Getting Ready for Twins

Expecting twins complicates decisions about what baby gear to get. Since as a parent of twins you'll have less time for each child, you may want more products to entertain a baby or otherwise save you trouble. But you don't really need two of everything, and you may be limited by space, finances, or both. You should make your decisions on the early side, too, because twins are often born early.

You may want to check whether your community has a Mothers of Twins Club (see Other Resources for New Parents, page 147). A local club could be a valuable resource for finding secondhand items in good condition.

FEEDING BY BREAST OR BOTTLE

. . . .

In addition to a basic breastfeeding guide such as *The Nursing Mother's Companion* (see The Parenting Bookshelf, page 141), you may want to read *Mothering Multiples: Breastfeeding & Caring for Twins and More* by Karen Kerkhoff Gromada (see The Parenting Bookshelf, page 141). This book is available from La Leche League.

Because half of them are born prematurely, twins are more likely to have trouble with breastfeeding at first. In this case, a rental breast pump is most efficient in establishing and maintaining milk production. Know ahead of time where to rent a pump (see page 32). Once the babies are nursing, pumping after most nursings can keep milk production high until the babies are gaining weight well without supplements.

Nursing both babies at once is a great time-saver. Nursing pillows made specifically for twins make it easier to do this. See Other Resources for New Parents (page 147) for information on ordering a twin nursing pillow.

It takes two arms to bottle-feed one baby, so formula-feeding parents of twins have a problem when both babies demand to be fed at the same time. You may hear about various bottle-propping devices, but all of these pose a risk of choking, in addition to depriving the baby of the warm bonding experience that feeding time normally provides. If a lack of help makes bottle propping a necessity, be sure to sit next to the self-feeding baby, and watch him closely. Some parents have used a twin nursing pillow to bottle-feed two babies at the same time.

SLEEPING ARRANGEMENTS

. . . .

This is another challenge for parents of twins, who handle it in a variety of ways. Many parents have their newborns sleep together in a cradle, a bedside sleeper, a crib, or a bassinet (larger-than-usual bassinets attached to play yards are a popular choice). Other parents have both babies sleep in the parental bed. Although newborn twins generally sleep better when snuggled side by side, some parents put their babies into separate beds right from the start.

As twins grow older, they may continue to sleep well together, or they may tend to wake each other up. Some parents start out with just one crib and wait to see how long the arrangement works. An inexpensive crib divider (see Other Resources for New Parents, page 147) can keep the babies from waking each other. If you think you want to buy two cribs at the start, ask whether a discount is available.

CLOTHING AND GEAR

Buying two of every piece of clothing cuts down substantially on how often laundry needs to be done. Most parents, however, can get by just fine with one and a half times the amount of clothing that they would buy for a single baby. Because twins often come early, buying some items in newborn sizes may be a good idea.

Buying two of every item of baby equipment—bouncer, swing, stationary entertainer, play yard, and so on—is expensive and for the most part unnecessary. Besides, all that gear would take up a tremendous amount of space in your home. You can buy a side-by-side bouncer for twins. This seat takes up less space than two separate bouncers, but some parents report that the twin bouncer was less useful than they had imagined. Some parents instead get a single bouncer and a swing, and switch the babies between the two when both are awake and in need of stimulation. Other parents invest in two swings, but these take up a great deal of space, and some babies don't like spending time in swings at all. Borrowing a swing or a bouncer in good condition may be the best option of all.

A front carrier, sling, or backpack is a good investment; it lets you have your arms free when you're carrying only one baby. Some parents carry one baby in a sling or other wearable carrier while pushing the other baby in a stroller. There is one soft carrier available for carrying two, or even three, babies at once (see Other Resources for New Parents, page 147).

Twin strollers are generally heavy and fairly expensive. Strollers for two come in two basic styles, tandem and side by side. Tandem strollers have one seat behind the other; these strollers may be more difficult to steer and to push over curbs, and usually only the back seat fully reclines. Many parents of twins prefer side-by-side strollers; these are easier to steer, and some have independently reclining seats. Side-by-side strollers come in a few styles, including umbrella and jogging as well as traditional. But side-by-side strollers may not fit through doorways or down narrow aisles; look for one measuring 30 inches wide or less if you will be going through doorways frequently. Side-by-sides also take up much more room when folded than tandem strollers do. A less expensive option for the early months is a stroller frame that accepts two car seats (see Other Resources for New Parents, page 147). Some parents have used a kit that allows for two inexpensive umbrella strollers to be joined together side by side, but they give this option mixed reviews. Such a makeshift side-by-side stroller may not be sturdy enough for regular use, although it can be helpful when traveling by air. Twin strollers in good condition can sometimes be purchased secondhand.

~≋~

Aside from buying and borrowing the things you will need for your twins, the most important thing to do ahead of time is to line up help for at least the first several weeks after your babies are born. If you are fortunate, friends and family members will be there for you and your partner. If they are not as available as you'd like, you might look into hiring someone to help with housekeeping and cooking.

CHAPTER 11

Baby-proofing and Other Safety Measures

Making your home safe for your child can be an overwhelming and expensive task. If money isn't a concern, you might consider hiring a specialist who will come to your home and do a complete childproofing job for you (see Other Resources for New Parents, page 147, for help in locating one). But keep in mind that you don't need to childproof the house completely before your baby is born. Many things can be worked on as your baby grows.

STAGE ONE

. . . .

These things should be done before your baby is born.

Monitor Smoke and Fumes

Make sure that you have smoke and carbon-monoxide detectors positioned in the necessary places around the house. Both kinds of detectors are available in hardware stores. Smoke detectors should go in each entry hall, in each hallway outside of bedrooms, in the kitchen, in the attic, in the basement, and in the garage. Smoke detectors should not be placed near air vents. If a smoke alarm goes off frequently in the kitchen or outside a bathroom, move the detector a little farther away instead of disabling it.

Carbon monoxide is an odorless, colorless gas that can be deadly if undetected. Symptoms of carbon-monoxide poisoning include headaches, dizziness, disorientation, nausea, and fatigue. When these symptoms are mild, they are often mistaken for the flu. Carbon-monoxide gas can come from gas-fired appliances, wood-burning furnaces, and fireplaces. To prevent carbon-monoxide poisoning:

◆ Place a carbon-monoxide detector on each level of your house or in areas suggested by the manufacturer.

◆ Never use your range or oven to heat your house, and never use a charcoal grill or hibachi in your house or garage.

◆ Do not keep a car running in a garage. Even if the garage doors are open, normal circulation will not provide enough fresh air to reliably prevent a dangerous buildup of carbon monoxide.

Check your smoke and carbon-monoxide detectors once a month, and replace the batteries once a year. Many people change the batteries when daylight savings time begins in October.

Prevent Burns

There are several things you can do to help keep your family and property safe from fire:

◆ Having a fire extinguisher in the kitchen is a good idea. Some people suggest having one on each level of the home. Look for type ABC extinguishers, which can be used for any type of fire.

◆ Make sure that emergency workers will be able to read the numbers of your address easily from the road.

◆ Placing a "tot finder" decal on the window of the baby's room or the outside lower corner of the nursery door might help firefighters locate your baby in a fire—but also inform would-be burglars or other intruders that the room is occupied by a defenseless child.

◆ Turn down the water heater to 120°F to prevent scalding. If for some reason you can't do this, consider installing a device on the bathtub faucet that will stop the flow of water if it exceeds 120°F.

Prevent Lead Poisoning

The number-one environmental health threat to children, lead can cause serious damage to the brain, nervous system, kidneys, and red blood cells. This damage can permanently lower a child's IQ. Lead poisoning can come from a variety of sources, including contaminated water and lead-based paint.

It has been estimated that the water supply in 20 percent of American homes contains a dangerous amount of lead—15 micrograms or more per liter. Lead can leach into tap water from lead pipes, connectors, and service lines and from bronze or brass faucets, which contain lead. Even copper pipes can have lead solder. Babies have been poisoned with lead from the water used to mix their formula. Lead levels in your drinking water are likely to be highest if:

◆ Your home has lead pipes or copper pipes with lead solder;

◆ Your house is less than five years old;

◆ You have soft water; or

◆ Water sits in the pipes for several hours.

Although many people believe that only older plumbing can cause lead contamination, buildings less than five years old most commonly have tap water with high levels of lead. This is because the solder from new pipes is not yet coated with mineral deposits. The only way to know the lead level in your household water is to have the water tested by a laboratory. Your local water or health department should be able either to provide this testing or to refer you to a qualified laboratory. According to the Environmental Protection Agency, the level should be no higher than 20 parts per billion.

Until you know the lead level in your water, buy bottled water or at least let your cold water run for two minutes or more before using it to mix formula (this flushing may not be effective in high-rise buildings). Never use water from the hot-water faucet for mixing formula, because hot water is likely to contain more lead. Boiling the water does not eliminate lead, but increases the level.

Lead-tainted paint chips and dust are very common in houses built before 1980, particularly on wood moldings around windows, floors, and doors, even if the moldings have been recently painted over. Some old pieces of furniture, including cribs and dressers, may be finished with lead-based paint or varnish. Lead test kits for old paint can be purchased from hardware stores, although some experts recommend having the testing done by a professional. See Other Resources for New Parents (page 147) for information on locating a lead specialist.

Design a Safe Nursery

The final area to be addressed before the baby is born is the nursery. Place the crib and changing table away from windows, wall hangings, cords, and heat sources. Bolt any high piece of furniture—a tall dresser, an armoire, or a bookcase—to the wall to prevent tipping. If you're planning to use a night-light, make sure the bulb is covered, because exposed bulbs can injure exploring babies. Or do without a night-light and use a wall or ceiling lamp with a low-wattage bulb or dimmer switch instead. A crib mobile should be hung out of a lying baby's reach and removed before the baby can stand to reach it.

STAGE TWO

. . . .

Once your baby begins rolling over, it is time for the second stage of childproofing. Go through your home room by room, looking around from a mobile baby's perspective. Many childproofing items can be found in hardware stores. For specialty items, see Other Resources for New Parents (page 147).

The Living Room

Televisions that are accessible should be secured to prevent them from falling. Place the TV in a cabinet that is secured to the wall, mount the TV directly on the wall, or secure it with furniture safety straps. TV and VCR guards are available to prevent babies from playing with knobs or inserting objects into the VCR opening.

Fireplace screens offer some protection from fireplaces and wood-burning stoves, but an installed fireplace railing is better. In any case, a baby or toddler should always be supervised when a fireplace or wood stove is in use. At other times, fireproof hearth padding can protect a baby from getting hurt on the hard surface of a hearth. Remove fireplace tools and the key to a gas fire starter.

Place floor lamps behind a barrier or remove them.

Babies often injure themselves on coffee tables. Installing soft plastic corner guards helps, but padding the entire table edge is better. Removable padding is commercially available, but it is easily removed by a baby as well as an adult. Some parents have discovered that sticky pipe wrap works better and costs less. If you don't want to disfigure your coffee table, it's best to remove it from the room.

CHILDPROOFING
CHECKLIST

· ·

☐ Firearms should be out of sight in a locked cabinet. Ammunition should be stored separately from the firearms.

☐ Houseplants should be out of reach. Poisonous plants, including philodendron, English ivy, azalea, and mistletoe, should be removed from your home. (Your local agricultural extension office or a nursery should be able to provide a list of poisonous plants.)

☐ Electrical outlets should be hidden by furniture or sliding outlet covers, which automatically close over the outlet when it is not in use. If you have outlets that are never used, you can screw on inexpensive blank plates. Use outlet plugs only if they fit so snugly that they require something thin and hard to pry them off. Easily removable outlet plugs not only attract little fingers to the outlet itself but are also a choking hazard.

☐ Other small items that may pose a choking hazard should be inaccessible. Anything that can fit into a toilet paper roll can choke a child.

☐ If furniture could tip over when climbed on by a child, it should be bolted to the wall.

☐ Doorknob covers are a good way to prevent toddlers from entering areas that are off-limits.

☐ Doors leading to the basement, garage, or outdoors should be secured with a high latch.

☐ Sliding glass doors should be locked and also secured by a rod or bar placed in the track. You can also buy a sliding door lock, which prevents the movable door from sliding over the stationary one.

☐ On balconies and stairways, babies can get stuck or fall between banisters, and toddlers may fall after climbing over them. Consider using a transparent banister shield, particularly if the vertical supports are spaced more than 4 inches apart.

☐ Gates can be used to prevent babies and toddlers from entering areas where there are pets or other hazards. Most of these gates are designed for openings of 28 to 32 inches, but some are made for larger openings, and some swing open so that parents can walk through. If you use a gate at the top of stairs, screw the frame into the wall; the gate should open away from the stairs. Pressure-mounted gates can be used in doorways between rooms on a single level. Wooden accordion-style gates are no longer recommended, because children can climb up on them.

☐ Accessible windows should be locked securely or fitted with a stopper or window guard so that they can be opened only about 4 inches. Window guards, which are mounted into the window frame, should be easily removable in case of fire.

☐ Furniture should not be placed in front of windows.

☐ Dangling cords of blinds or shades should be cut short or kept out of a child's reach.

☐ Electrical cords from lamps, televisions, appliances, and computers should be placed behind or under furniture. Outlet strips should be fitted with childproof covers. Flexible tubing is available for covering multiple cords at once.

☐ Pet food and water bowls and litter boxes should be inaccessible.

☐ No dog should ever be left alone with a baby; even dogs with no history of violence have attacked newborns, sometimes when the babies were in swings. Some families have hired trainers to make sure their dogs will behave well around their babies. Pet gates may be helpful, too.

☐ Radiators and other heat sources should be inaccessible.

The Kitchen

Toxic items should be completely out of reach or under lock and key. Everyday dishwashing items can remain under the sink, secured by a cabinet lock. Drawers containing sharp items can be secured with drawer latches. Put a latch on the drawer that holds plastic bags and plastic wrap, too.

Among kitchen stoves, the most dangerous are the ones that look like countertops even when they are turned on. You can either remove the stove knobs and store them until needed or fit them with knob covers. When you are cooking and need only one or two burners at a time, use the back ones, and always turn the pot handles inward. Use built-in appliance locks on ovens, dishwashers, and trash compactors when these are not in use. If your appliances don't have built-in locks, buy appliance latches for them. These latches also work for ovens, refrigerators, and freezers. Move chairs and stools away from countertops and stoves.

The Bathroom

Even if you try to keep bathrooms off-limits with a doorknob cover or doorway gate, it's wise to use a toilet-seat lock. Pad the bathtub spout with a cover to protect against burns and bumps. Store medicines, vitamins, and toiletries in locked cabinets, and keep electrical items in a secure place.

The Yard

Your yard should be fenced. If your porch or deck has rails spaced more than 4 inches apart, they should be covered by a mesh railing guard. Any water containers should be kept empty.

The most dangerous yard feature is a pool, spa, or pond. It should be fenced apart from any area accessible by children, with a self-closing gate and a latch that is out of reach. If you have an above-ground pool, make the stairs inaccessible or remove them when the pool is not in use. Pool covers and underwater alarms provide additional safety.

There are a few more measures you can take to keep your baby alive and well. If you've never taken first-aid and CPR classes, try to do this during the latter part of pregnancy. Post emergency telephone numbers, including poison control and the baby's doctor, near your telephone. Get the first-aid items listed in chapter 6, and keep them somewhere handy in your home. And remember that, no matter how well you prepare your home, there is no substitute for keeping a watchful eye on your baby.

CHAPTER 12

Daycare Options

I f both you and your partner need to return to work after the birth of your child, the search for daycare can be very stressful. If you're very lucky, you may have family members or friends who can help care for your baby. Even if you do, you may need to think hard about what kind of care you want and whether you can afford it. This chapter outlines some choices.

RELATIVES AS CARE PROVIDERS

. . . .

About 20 percent of young children of working parents are cared for by family members, usually a parent, sister, aunt, or cousin of one of the baby's parents. Probably no other type of child care can offer as much peace of mind: The provider really cares about your child's well-being; your baby is in a home—the relative's if not your own—rather than in an institution; and he is likely to get plenty of one-on-one attention. With fewer children around, he'll probably get sick less often than he would in a daycare center. Lastly, relatives usually come cheaper than other child-care providers.

It may be hard, though, to become the employer of a family member. If you and your relative disagree in your philosophies about feeding, sleep, and other matters, you may have a hard time communicating your desires, especially if the relative insists on working for free. In this case, you'll want to show as much appreciation as you can while gently explaining your preferences.

Older relatives may take on more than they really should. Some may do well with an infant but lack the stamina to care for an active toddler. Or perhaps one child is fine, but a second may require more energy than Grandma has. If you sense that your relative is having difficulty keeping your child entertained or safe from dangerous situations, it may be time to look for another care provider.

Your relative may prefer to care for your child in her own home, or she may be happy to come to yours. Whatever works best for the provider is probably best for everyone. She may feel more comfortable and less inconvenienced in her own home, or she may prefer your house because it is childproofed and fully equipped for the baby.

NANNIES

. . . .

A professional child-care provider who supervises children in the family home, a nanny may live and eat in the home or commute. Many nannies are trained in child care and child development; others have learned through experience.

Although a nanny may be the most expensive care provider, there are many advantages to hiring one. A nanny provides one-on-one attention, and babies who stay home with few or no other children are exposed to fewer illnesses. A nanny usually offers scheduling flexibility; she may be willing to work as many as 50 hours per week. Although her priority will be the children, she may happily take on other household duties, such as running errands, cooking, and light housekeeping. Unlike an au pair, who must return to her home country after one year, a nanny may stay with the family indefinitely.

There are disadvantages to hiring a nanny, of course. She must be paid decent wages, and she will probably expect fringe benefits such as paid vacation and health insurance. Live-in nannies earn about $250 to $500 per week, commuting nannies at least $10 per hour in urban areas and $8 per hour elsewhere. There are also tax requirements when you hire a nanny. Lastly, in the care of a nanny your child may spend less time socializing with other children than you'd like.

One way to find a nanny is through a nanny-referral agency. These agencies interview the family, recruit candidates, check their employment and personal references, and refer finalists to the family. After the family interviews a candidate they like, the agency makes the job offer and helps the family write a work contract. The agency then orders a background check and advises the family on salary and tax issues. The agency collects its fee, usually between $1,500 and $5,000, when the nanny starts work. Typically, this fee includes a one-year guarantee.

There are Internet-based nanny-referral services, too. These charge less than traditional agencies but also provide less service. Through a Web site, you can preview unscreened candidates. If you think there is a likely candidate in the pool, you pay a subscription fee of about $200 to $350. Then you receive information about how to contact the candidates. You do all of the screening yourself, including checking employment and personal references. You also make the job offer and write a work agreement yourself, although the Web site may have tools to help with these and other matters, such as payroll taxes and insurance. Through the Web site, you then order a background check, the fee for which may be included in the subscription cost.

Many families recruit and hire nannies on their own. Advertisements in newspapers, churches, senior centers, and schools should include basic requirements, including experience, workdays and hours, driving requirements, references, and when to call. The nanny should have experience in caring for infants. You may also require that she speak English, refrain from smoking, and have CPR certification. When candidates call, have a list of basic questions ready, and don't forget to ask for references. Check the references before scheduling an interview. Before you offer someone the job, you might have a background check done; this costs from $50 to $150. Write an agreement outlining duties and compensation. Make sure you know how to deal with payroll tax, medical insurance obligations, and workers' compensation. If the nanny will be driving the family vehicle, add her to your automobile insurance policy.

Regardless of how you go about finding a nanny, the interview is an important chance to learn about the candidate. Don't make the mistake of talking too much yourself, or of asking questions that require only a yes or no answer. You'll find out more about the candidate with open-ended questions like these:

◆ Tell me about your last child-care job. Why did you leave it?

◆ What do you like best about working with children?

- What is the most difficult part of being a nanny?
- Tell me about the most difficult experience you've had in caring for children. How did you resolve it?
- Tell me about your childhood.
- How were you disciplined? How would you (or how did you) discipline your own children?
- Tell me about your last three employers. What did you like and dislike about each of them?
- How do you handle a crying baby?
- What questions do you have for me?

After the interview, listen to your instincts. If you have any nagging doubts, move on to another candidate.

Some families decide to share a nanny. This arrangement can work well as long as the families agree on a person to hire, pay and contract details, and the use of one home or the other. The parents must be sure that they share similar views about the children's activities, discipline, and feeding, and they should communicate continually about day-to-day problems. When the families work well together, sharing a nanny saves them money, provides each child with a regular playmate, and makes it easier to find a substitute when the nanny is unavailable.

AU PAIRS

An au pair is a foreign student between 18 and 26 years old who enters the United States to live with an American family and care for its children for a year. Work hours are limited to 10 per day and 45 per week, and au pairs are not to assume household duties other than caring for children. Besides providing child care, the au pair must complete six semester hours of college classes.

The Au Pair Program was established in 1986 to provide educational and cultural exchange opportunities with a component of family child care. Sponsoring organizations place au pairs with families according to rules established by the U.S. Department of State. An au pair may come from any country with which the United States has diplomatic relations. A participant must have a secondary-school diploma and speak English proficiently.

Although she is not a professional child-care provider, an au pair has basic training. Before she is placed with a family, she receives at least eight hours of child-safety instruction, including CPR, and at least 24 hours of child-development instruction. If she will be responsible for children under the age of two, she must document that she has cared for children for at least 200 hours. Except when a parent or other adult is in the home, she may not care for infants under three months of age.

The French term *au pair,* meaning "on par," implies that the student should be treated as a family member. All her meals and a private room must be provided. The family must assist with enrolling her in classes and transporting her to them. The family also pays a $500 educational allowance. The au pair must get one and a half days off each week, one weekend off each month, and two weeks of paid vacation.

An au pair comes much cheaper than a nanny: The average cost for a year is $13,000. This includes a weekly stipend, the educational allowance, and a fee for the sponsoring organization. There are no employment taxes to pay.

A sponsoring organization does quite a lot to earn its fee. It screens prospective au pairs and helps match them to families. It conducts background investigations and interviews au pairs to assess their English proficiency and suitability for providing child care. The organization also interviews host families to make sure they have the means to pay for an au pair and can manage dealing with an international student. The sponsoring organization provides the au pair with a detailed profile of the family, the community, and available educational programs, and arranges for the au pair's child-safety and child-development instruction. Every month, the organization monitors the ongoing relationship between the family and the au pair through regional counselors.

Host parents interview au pair candidates by phone before making a final decision. A written agreement outlining the responsibilities of both parties must be signed by the au pair and the parents.

Many organizations are authorized by the U.S. Department of State to participate in the Au Pair Program. Although all are required to follow the guidelines set up by the U.S. government, each organization interprets the guidelines a little differently. You can find a list of authorized organizations on the Web site of the International Au Pair Association, www.iapa.org.

The biggest disadvantage to hiring an au pair may be that she must return to her home country at the end of the year. This may be especially difficult for the children, if they have become very attached to her.

FAMILY
DAYCARE

. . . .

A popular child-care option is small-group daycare in a family home. Besides providing a homey atmosphere, family daycare usually costs less than one-on-one care and often offers flexible hours. On the downside, few family daycare providers have formal education in child development, not all states require licensed providers to take basic health and safety courses, and not all providers are licensed. Also, if the provider gets sick or takes a vacation, you may have to find another, temporary child-care arrangement.

Family daycare providers are required to be licensed by the state unless the provider is caring only for her own children and those of one other family. Despite the law, many providers who should be licensed aren't. You can get a list of licensed family daycare providers from your local Child Care Resource Center, which you can find by contacting Child Care Aware (800-424-2246, www.childcareaware.org).

Licensing requirements differ from state to state. Child Care Aware can tell you exactly what the requirements are in your state. Generally, a license ensures minimal standards but not high-quality care. Some family daycare providers take their work seriously enough to become accredited by the National Association for Family Child Care. Find out whether a provider is accredited and exactly what this accreditation means by checking the association's Web site, www.nafcc.org, or by telephoning 800-359-3817.

When you find a family daycare provider with an opening, you will want to pay the home a visit. Try to schedule your visit for a time when the children are not napping. Find out how many infants there are, and whether this number meets the provider's license specifications. Assess the environment. Is the home clean? Is there enough space for exploring? Does television seem to be the main entertainment? Are there washable, age-appropriate toys? Is the home childproofed?

Watch how the provider interacts with the children. Does she hold and talk with the babies, or do they seem to spend much of their time in swings, car seats, or cribs? Does she respond to the babies and toddlers immediately when they cry, and hold them for bottle feedings? Does she interact continuously with the children or just watch them? To learn more about the provider, ask open-ended questions, such as these:

- Why did you become a daycare provider?
- What do you like best about working with children?
- What is the hardest part of being a daycare provider?
- Tell me about the most difficult experience you've had in caring for children in your home. How did you resolve it?
- How were you disciplined when you were a child? How do you (or how did you) discipline your own children?
- What health, safety, or child-development classes have you attended?
- How do you handle a crying baby?
- How do you feel about feeding and napping schedules?

◆ How do you feel about feeding expressed breast milk?

◆ What questions do you have for me?

If you feel comfortable with the provider, ask about her policies, including those regarding hours, fees, and sickness. How are vacations handled, both yours and hers? Will you need to provide diapers for your baby? Ask for the names and telephone numbers of three families whose babies the provider has cared for. Call them all to ask about their experience with this family daycare provider.

DAYCARE CENTERS

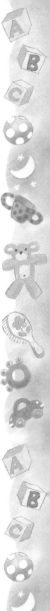

Publicly funded, private, or associated with a religious group, these centers may or may not accept infants. Because the best centers often have waiting lists, you may need to start investigating and touring centers months before your baby is due.

Most states require that centers caring for more than 12 children be licensed. Depending on the state, the license may mean only that the center meets very basic standards. You can find out your state's licensing requirements and get a list of licensed centers from your local Child Care Resource Center, which you can find by contacting Child Care Aware (800-424-2246, www.childcareaware.org). Some daycare centers meet the strict standards of the National Association for the Education of Young Children. To find out which local centers have received accreditation from the association, consult its Web site, www.naeyc.org, or telephone 800-424-2460.

Child-care centers offer many advantages over other types of child care. Overseen by a director, the staff typically has had formal instruction in child development. If one staff member is sick or takes a vacation, others fill in. Daycare centers offer a wide variety of activities and plenty of opportunity for interaction with other children. Using a daycare center is usually less expensive than hiring a nanny or getting an au pair.

Daycare centers have serious disadvantages, though. Your child will probably get much less personal attention in a center than he would from an in-home provider. He will be more often exposed to infectious diseases. This means he will be likelier to get sick himself, and when he does you will have to arrange for other care. Daycare centers usually have strict hours, so you could end up paying late fees whenever you run late.

When you visit a daycare center, pay attention to numbers. Find out how many infants are cared for at the facility, and make sure the ratio of infants to care providers is no more than three to one. Check that no more than six infants share a room, and that toddlers and preschoolers are cared for in rooms separate from the babies. Make sure each baby has his own crib.

Assess the environment. Is the center clean and spacious? Are there washable, age-appropriate toys? Is the diaper-changing area clean and near a sink? Does the infant area seem to be childproof?

Observe interactions between children and providers. Are infants under constant observation? Do staff members hold and talk to them, or do the babies spend much of their time in swings, car seats, or cribs? Does a provider respond immediately when a baby cries? Are babies held for all of their bottle feedings?

Interview both the director and the staff member(s) who would care for your baby. Ask about the center's policies. Does each staff member care for the same babies every day? Is there a feeding and napping schedule that must be adhered to? Are diapers provided? Is the center willing to store your breast milk and feed it to your baby? Ask about matters such as hours and fees, and get the names and phone numbers of three families who have had infants at the center. Call them all to ask about their experiences.

After you've gone through an intensive selection process, you may feel confident that you've found the best daycare possible for your baby. But don't stop watching and asking questions. You must continuously monitor the daycare setting and provider to ensure a happy, healthy experience for your child.

The Parenting Bookshelf

These are the books I most often recommend to expectant parents.

Balaskas, Janet. *Active Birth: The New Approach to Giving Birth Naturally,* rev. ed. Boston: The Harvard Common Press, 1992.

This book encourages women to take control of their childbirth experience by participating actively in their delivery. The author suggests that mothers follow their own instincts, move freely, and find comfortable, effective positions for labor and delivery.

Brazelton, T. Berry. *Touchpoints: Your Child's Emotional and Behavioral Development.* Cambridge, Mass.: Perseus Books, 1992.

Touchpoints presents the basic stages of early childhood development and explores the important role of each family member in a child's life. Dr. Brazelton provides the kindly, reassuring approach you might expect from your child's own pediatrician.

Gromada, Karen Kerkhoff. *Mothering Multiples: Breastfeeding & Caring for Twins or More,* rev. ed. Schaumburg, Ill.: La Leche League International, 1999.

Gromada is a perinatal nurse and a board-certified lactation consultant who has worked with hundreds of mothers of multiples. The book is full of practical information about prenatal care, pregnancy, preterm labor, birth, diet, milk expression, and the daily care of more than one baby.

Huggins, Kathleen. *The Nursing Mother's Companion,* 5th ed. Boston: The Harvard Common Press, 2005.

The Nursing Mother's Companion is a comprehensive, practical guide for easy reference throughout the nursing period. The first part of the book provides basic information about the breast, preparation for nursing, and nursing during the first week after baby's birth; the remainder is for reading as the baby and nursing relationship grow and develop from the first week through toddlerhood. Chapters called Survival Guides enable mothers to identify and resolve nursing problems as quickly as possible.

Huggins, Kathleen, and Linda Ziedrich. *The Nursing Mother's Guide to Weaning.* Boston: The Harvard Common Press, 1994.

This book not only provides how-to advice for weaning a baby, toddler, or older child, but also explains how to overcome many difficulties that may cause mothers to initiate weaning prematurely. The book includes a lively history of weaning in Western societies.

Karp, Harvey. *The Happiest Baby on the Block: The New Way to Calm Crying and Help Your Baby Sleep Longer.* New York: Bantam Books, 2002.

Pediatrician Karp offers parents of newborns a new method to help calm and soothe their crying infants.

Kleiman, Karen R., and Valerie D. Raskin. *This Isn't What I Expected: Overcoming Postpartum Depression.* New York: Bantam Books, 1994.

In this thorough guide to postpartum emotional problems and their treatment, the authors debunk the myths surrounding postpartum depression and provide compassionate support and solid advice for women who struggle with this difficult condition.

Lothian, Judith, and Charlotte DeVries. *The Official Lamaze Guide: Giving Birth with Confidence.* New York: Meadowbrook Press, 2005.

The authors, both Lamaze childbirth educators, provide clear, solid evidence that common medical interventions during labor and delivery put both mother and baby at greater risk than does "normal" childbirth. Lothian and DeVries bring decades of experience backed by scientific research to support their advice on the best ways to prepare for childbirth.

Pantley, Elizabeth. *The No-Cry Sleep Solution: Gentle Ways to Help Your Baby Sleep Through the Night.* Chicago: Contemporary Books, 2002.

Pantley teaches parents, step by step, how to help their babies learn to fall asleep without "crying it out," and how to help them stay asleep through the night, whether in a crib or the family bed. Pantley offers real-life answers to one of the most challenging situations that parents face.

Rozario, Diane. *The Immunization Resource Guide: Where to Find Answers to All Your Questions about Childhood Immunizations.* Burlington, Iowa: Patter Publications, 2000.

Rosario reviews books and periodicals covering all aspects of childhood immunizations. Topics include vaccines and the immune system, the history of vaccination, the DTP vaccine, obtaining legal exemptions from mandated vaccinations, adverse reactions, and national, state, and local vaccine support groups.

Satter, Ellyn. *Child of Mine: Feeding with Love and Good Sense.* Boulder, Colo.: Bull Publishing, 2000.

In this wonderful book about nutrition for infants and young children, Satter offers basic information about breastfeeding, bottle-feeding, the transition to solid food, and normal growth from infancy through preschool.

Sears, William, and Martha Sears. *The Baby Book: Everything You Need to Know About Your Baby from Birth to Age Two,* 2nd ed. Boston: Little, Brown, 2003.

The Baby Book focuses on the essential needs of babies—eating, sleeping, development, health, and comfort—as it addresses the questions of greatest concern to parents.

Simkin, Penny. *The Birth Partner: Everything You Need to Know to Help a Woman Through Childbirth,* 2nd. ed. Boston: The Harvard Common Press, 2001.

This is the definitive guide for preparing to help a woman through childbirth and the essential manual to have at hand during the event.

Simkin, Penny, Janet Whalley, and Ann Keppler. *Pregnancy, Childbirth, and the Newborn: The Complete Guide,* rev. ed. New York: Meadowbrook Press, 2001.

This book covers prenatal care, labor support techniques, birth plans, medical interventions, relaxation, and postpartum adjustment, with a strong emphasis on parental choice.

Other Resources for New Parents

··

LABOR AND DELIVERY SUPPORT

Childbirth Instructors

Lamaze International
800-368-4404
www.lamaze.org

Bradley Method of Natural
 Childbirth
800-4-A-BIRTH
www.bradleybirth.com

International Childbirth
 Education Association
952-854-8660
www.icea.org

Professional Birth Assistants

Childbirth and Postpartum
 Professional Association
888-MY-CAPPA
www.cappa.net

DONA (Doulas of North
 America) International
888-788-DONA
www.dona.org

International Childbirth
 Education Association
952-854-8660
www.icea.org

Birthing Pools

YourWaterBirth.com
509-764-2992
www.yourwaterbirth.com

Aqua Doula
800-275-6144
www.aquadoula.com

Birthing Balls

Birth with Sol
800-9-FOR-SOL
www.birthwithsol.com

The Doula Shop
www.doulashop.com

POSTPARTUM SUPPORT

Childbirth and Postpartum
 Professional Association
888-MY-CAPPA
www.cappa.net

DONA (Doulas of North
 America) International
888-788-DONA
www.dona.org

National Association of
 Postpartum Care Services
800-453-6852
www.napcs.org

BREASTFEEDING SUPPORT

La Leche League International
847-519-7730
www.lalecheleague.org

International Lactation
   Consultant Association
919-861-5577
www.ilca.org

BREASTFEEDING EQUIPMENT

Breast Pump Rental

Medela
800-435-8316
www.medela.com

Hollister
800-323-4060
www.hollister.com/us

Nursing Stools

Medela
800-435-8316
www.medela.com

Lansinoh Nursing Pads

Lansinoh pads are available at Albertsons, Safeway, Target, Wal-Mart, and numerous drugstore chains such as Rite-Aid, Walgreens, and CVS.

Nursing Pillow

My Brest Friend
www.mybrestfriend.com
Available at BabiesRUs, Burlington Coat Factory, and other stores.

Milk Storage Bottles and Bags

Mother's Milk Mate Storage
   Bottles
Available through La Leche League (847-519-7730; www.lalecheleague.org).

MOM's Bags
888-666-7224
www.momsboutique.com

Medela Milk Bags
800-435-8316
www.medela.com

BABY BEDS AND CARRIERS

Amby Baby Hammock
866-519-BABY
www.ambybaby.com
Provides a gentle rocking motion to help babies sleep better and longer.

Deluxe Snuggle Nest
877-810-9350
www.snugglenest.com
A padded plastic baby bed to use in the parents' bed.

Baby Carriers

Baby Björn
877-242-5676
www.babybjorn.com

Ergo Baby Carrier
888-416-4888
www.ergobabycarrier.com

RESOURCES FOR PARENTS OF TWINS

Mothers of Twins Clubs
877-540-2200
www.nomotc.org

Products for Twins

These items are available from Double Blessings (800-584-TWIN, www.doubleblessings.com) and other Internet vendors.

EZ-2-Nurse Twins nursing pillow

MaxiMom baby carrier
A unique soft carrier that enables parents to carry twins or even triplets.

Leachco Crib Spacer
Divides a crib into two small beds.

Baby Trend Double Snap N Go stroller frame
Attach two infant car seats to make an inexpensive stroller.

CHILD-CARE CENTER LICENSING INFORMATION

Child Care Aware
800-424-2246
www.childcareaware.org

CHILD SAFETY INFORMATION AND EQUIPMENT

Car Seat Safety Information

National Highway Traffic
 Safety Administration
888-327-4236
www.nhtsa.dot.gov
Information on car-seat recalls and car-seat inspection locations.

Home Safety Experts

InfantHouse.Com
866-INFANT-5
www.infanthouse.com

Safe & Sound
610-539-7020
www.123safe.com

Lead Testing

National Lead Information
 Center
800-424-5323
www.epa.gov/lead/nlic.htm

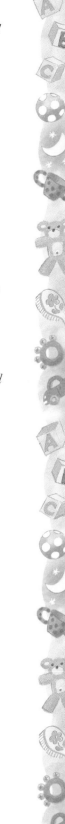

Index

Doctors' Visits

Postpartum Helpers

Baby Gift Wish List

_____

_____

_____

_____

_____

_____

_____

_____

_____

_____

_____

_____

_____

_____

_____

_____

_____

_____

_____

_____

_____

_____

_____

Gift Log

Other Child Care and Parenting Books
from The Harvard Common Press

Harvard Common Press books are available wherever books are sold. If you have any questions or are interested in resale of Harvard Common Press books, please call 617-423-5803 or 888-657-3755. To learn more about Harvard Common Press parenting titles, please visit our Web site: www.harvardcommonpress.com.

THE NURSING MOTHER'S COMPANION
20th Anniversary Edition
by Kathleen Huggins, R.N., M.S.
$14.95 paperback, ISBN 1-55832-304-X

The fifth edition of this best-selling, widely acclaimed guide for nursing mothers has been completely revised and updated. In addition to covering all the basics of breastfeeding, the book includes an extensive index on the safety of drugs during breastfeeding and "survival guide" sections to help nursing mothers quickly identify and solve problems during each stage of breastfeeding.

THE NURSING MOTHER'S GUIDE TO WEANING
by Kathleen Huggins, R.N., M.S., and Linda Ziedrich
$11.95 paperback, ISBN 1-55832-065-2

Provides invaluable advice on a subject that has caused distress for countless mothers—when and how to wean—with guidance on the safest, least stressful ways to bring breastfeeding to a gentle close at every age, from early infancy through toddlerhood and beyond.

NURSING MOTHER, WORKING MOTHER
THE ESSENTIAL GUIDE FOR BREASTFEEDING
AND STAYING CLOSE TO YOUR BABY
AFTER YOU RETURN TO WORK
by Gale Pryor
$12.95 paperback, ISBN 1-55832-117-9

With straightforward information and an encouraging tone, Pryor advises working mothers who want to continue breastfeeding on everything from how to simplify life at home to how to maintain one's milk supply, pump breast milk at work, and store and transport breast milk safely and conveniently.

25 THINGS EVERY NEW MOTHER SHOULD KNOW
by Martha Sears, R.N., with William Sears, M.D.
$12.95 hardcover, ISBN 1-55832-315-5

America's top baby-care experts offer a collection of 25 insightful and timeless tips for new mothers to help them acclimate to and enjoy their new role as parents.

FATHER'S FIRST STEPS
25 THINGS EVERY NEW DAD SHOULD KNOW
by Robert W. Sears, M.D., and James M. Sears, M.D.
$12.95 hardcover, ISBN 1-55832-335-X

The companion book to 25 *Things Every New Mother Should Know* offers invaluable, practical tips for new dads. The authors are fathers, pediatricians, and sons of America's top baby-care experts, William and Martha Sears.

NINE MONTHS AND A DAY
A PREGNANCY AND BIRTH COMPANION
by Adrienne B. Lieberman and Linda Hughey Holt, M.D.
$10.95 paperback, ISBN 1-55832-318-X

This concise yet thorough guide to pregnancy and delivery offers all the essential information a mom-to-be will want at her fingertips, including checklists of questions for each stage of pregnancy, tips for easing the aches and pains of pregnancy, and lists of what to have in the house for baby's homecoming.

HELLO, MY NAME IS . . .
A GUIDE TO NAMING YOUR BABY
by Jeff, Truman, and Walker Bradley
$14.95 paperback, ISBN 1-55832-280-9

Find the perfect name for baby in this inspiring collection of both traditional and unique choices and amusing naming lore.

THE BIRTH PARTNER
EVERYTHING YOU NEED TO KNOW TO HELP
A WOMAN THROUGH CHILDBIRTH
Second Edition
by Penny Simkin, P.T.
$14.95 paperback, ISBN 1-55832-195-0

This comprehensive guide to birth provides advice for the mother's chief helper, whether that person is her mate, friend, or relative. The book includes positions, breathing patterns, and other comfort measures for labor; the intended effects and side effects of various pain medications; problems that may arise in labor and obstetric interventions; and postpartum care of the mother and baby. Each chapter contains plentiful concrete advice on how the helper can be most helpful.

THE PREEMIE PARENTS' COMPANION
THE ESSENTIAL GUIDE TO CARING FOR YOUR PREMATURE BABY IN THE
HOSPITAL, AT HOME, AND THROUGH THE FIRST YEARS
by Susan L. Madden, M.S.
$16.95 paperback, ISBN 1-55832-135-7

In a warm and supportive manner, Madden helps parents of premature babies
overcome their uncertainty and actively participate in their baby's care both in
the hospital and at home, through the developmentally crucial first years.

ACTIVE BIRTH
THE NEW APPROACH TO GIVING BIRTH NATURALLY
Revised Edition
by Janet Balaskas
$14.95 paperback, ISBN 1-55832-038-5

This important resource encourages women to become active participants in
childbirth, with information on yoga-based exercises for pregnancy, effective
positions and movements for labor at home or in the hospital, and postpartum
exercises for recovery after birth.

A GOOD BIRTH, A SAFE BIRTH
CHOOSING AND HAVING THE CHILDBIRTH EXPERIENCE YOU WANT
Third Revised Edition
by Diana Korte and Roberta Scaer
$15.95 paperback, ISBN 1-55832-041-5

This invaluable reference provides detailed information about childbirth
options, with advice on finding an appropriate doctor and hospital, questions
women can ask to help them have the kind of childbirth experience they want,
the benefits and drawbacks of medications during labor, and more.